Reshaping Life

RESHAPING
LIFE
KEY ISSUES
IN
GENETIC ENGINEERING

G. J. V. NOSSAL

MELBOURNE UNIVERSITY PRESS

First published 1984
Reprinted 1985
Printed in Australia by
The Dominion Press-Hedges & Bell, Victoria, for
Melbourne University Press, Carlton, Victoria 3053

National Library of Australia Cataloguing-in-Publication entry

Nossal, G. J. V. (Gustav Joseph Victor), 1931 –
    Reshaping life.
    Bibliography.
    Includes index.
    Simultaneously published: Cambridge, Cambridgeshire:
    Cambridge University Press.
    ISBN 0 522 84278 X.

    1. Genetic engineering. I. Title.

575.1

For my colleagues at The Walter and Eliza Hall
Institute of Medical Research – young and old –
who are my best teachers.

By the same author:

Antibodies and Immunity

Antigens, Lymphoid Cells and the Immune Response (with G. L. Ada)

Medical Science and Human Goals

Nature's Defences – New Frontiers of Vaccine Research

Contents

Contents

Contents

Contents

Illustrations

Acknowledgements

The adventure of learning about genetic engineering I owe to my colleagues at The Walter and Eliza Hall Institute, who have contributed so notably to the field's progress. Rosalind Brown was a gentle and persuasive critic and also helped greatly with the Glossary and Index. Andrew Abbot, Richard Mahony and Sonya Belan worked wonders with the illustrations, and the typing staff of The Walter and Eliza Hall Institute, under the leadership of Peta McGovern, were (as usual) extraordinarily speedy and effective.

This is Publication Number 3333 from the Hall Institute. My own research has been supported by The National Health and Medical Research Council, Canberra, Australia, by Grant Number AI-03958 from the National Institute for Allergy and Infectious Diseases, United States Public Health Service, and by generous private donors to the Hall Institute.

G. J. V. Nossal
Melbourne
May 1984

1
The Genie is out of the Bottle

When historians look back on the twentieth century, they will conclude that its first half was shaped by the physical sciences but its second by biology. The first half of the century brought the revolution in transportation, communications, mass production technology and the beginnings of the computer age. It also ushered in nuclear weapons and an irrevocable change in the nature of warfare. All these changes and many more rested on physics and chemistry. Biological science, too, was stirring over those decades. The development of vaccines and antibiotics and early harbingers of the green revolution represented proud achievements. Yet the public preoccupation with the physical sciences and technologies, and the immense upheavals in man's estate which these brought, meant that biology and medicine could only move to centre stage somewhat later. Moreover, the intricacies of living structures are such that their deepest secrets could only be revealed after the physical sciences had produced the tools—electron microscopes, radioisotopes, chemical analysers—required for penetrating study. Accordingly, it is only now that the fruits of biological science have jostled their way to the front pages.

In the eye of the storm we find DNA. This long but essentially rather simple molecule is the key to the puzzle of life. It embodies what each biological species looks like, how long it lives, what the limits of its potential are. It specifies in the minutest detail what each plant or animal, and indeed each cell in each plant or animal, can do. For this reason DNA has been termed the thread of life; the progressive elucidation of its structure and function have rightly been biology's central preoccupation since 1950. If this is so, why the unique excitement about DNA over the last few years? What is so new, so special?

For a quarter of a century between 1950 and 1975, DNA was

thought by most scientists to be like a remote dictator within a fortified stronghold—inviolate, sacrosanct, issuing orders but itself still and unchanging. Then came the genetic engineers, and, with a speed that was truly breathtaking, they changed the image of DNA. They made it accessible to a whole new generation of investigators, unafraid of its big reputation. DNA contains the genes, the fundamental units of inheritance, the blueprints for the cell's work. Genetic engineers split DNA open, cut out individual genes, transplanted them into bacteria or other cells, reproduced them a billion times. They created hybrids in the test tube unlike anything that three and a half billion years of evolution had accomplished. Within less than a decade, it became clear that genetic engineering and related technologies represented the biggest single advance in the life sciences this century. It held the key to a deeper understanding of human diseases, including cancer. It offered glittering prizes to industry. It promised to free agriculture from constraining requirements for fertilizers and pesticides. There seemed no limits to what the genetic engineers would dare. The genie was out of the bottle.

Unlike the atomic age, which was born in secrecy during a world war, the DNA age has begun amidst the fiercest blaze of publicity. An unprecedented act of global self-censorship by the scientific community, which in 1974 placed a brief moratorium on genetic engineering research until potential hazards could be assessed, was predictably misinterpreted by society. Scaremongers abounded, and much of the public debate created more heat than light. In the event, patience and sanity prevailed and the research was resumed in 1975 under stringent safeguards that, with hindsight, proved unnecessarily elaborate. It is to the enduring credit of both scientists and their critics that the legislative framework permitting continued advance relied more on regulatory guidelines than on proscriptions and sanctions. As a result, genetic engineering research has infiltrated virtually every nook and cranny of bio-medicine. The DNA industry exists undeterred by a lake of red ink. Philosophers and jurists have discovered a new cause. Large multinational pharmaceutical firms are re-examining their research and development strategy. Governments are groping for novel schemes to nurture what they hope will be a source of employment and export income. Above all, the journalists of both print and electronic media have joyously embraced the new wonder as the quintessential source of a continuous stream of 'breakthroughs' and 'cures'.

Why, then, another book on genetic engineering? What could possibly remain to be said? The need for a particular type of statement dawned on me gradually. In the normal course of work as Director of a large medical research institute I interact with many segments of society. Many of my lay contacts display a lively interest in research. However, I had been so saturated with gaudy press releases on the one hand, and weighty techni-cal tomes on the other, that I had missed a central point about genetic engineering. Those of us within science who have wit-nessed the birth of this amazing development; those of us who sit on the endless Government committees and write the dry technical reports; even those of us who honestly strive to brief the young journalist on his first scientific assignment; we have all been too close to the problem. We have forgotten how alien the concepts of genes and cells and molecules are to the layman. We use our own special language, unconsciously slipping in unfamiliar technical terms, and we soon lose even a hard-working listener. Yet it is vitally important that the potential and also the limitations of genetic engineering be made access-ible to a wide public, the more so as its central concepts are really simple. Therefore, the aim of this book is to present the essential elements of genetic engineering within a slim volume in a manner requiring no background in biology and for a readership with no technical expertise in the field. The target audience includes decision-makers at many levels; politicians, financiers and industrialists, community leaders, academics in non-biological fields. I also hope to stimulate a diversity of people from all walks of life interested in informing themselves about a key development which, slowly but surely, will reshape many aspects of their children's lives. My greatest wish is to stir the interest of the young, for example the school leaver ponder-ing a career, so that the fascination of the field may tempt a few to become its future devotees.

Genetic engineering cannot be intelligently approached with-out some reference to basic biology. In the next chapter the bare bones of biological organization will be described. Following that, we discuss how genetic engineering works. These two chapters get us over the toughest hurdles, because thereafter we deal with practical fruits and social implications of this extra-ordinary turning point in mankind's affairs. I have no illusions about the effort which will be required by non-scientific readers to follow Chapters 2 and 3. If a quick scan of them seems formidably daunting to you, I suggest you skip over them and go straight to Chapter 4. This explains how hormones and other human proteins of use in the treatment of serious diseases can be mass-produced by genetic engineering. Chapter 5 describes how purified genes can help to diagnose hereditary and other diseases, and Chapter 6 goes on to speculate about how, in the future, good genes might be able to be substituted for bad ones right within the body of the patient. Chapter 7 examines some disease problems of the tropical developing countries, with special reference to new vaccines made through genetic engineering. Chapters 8 and 9 look at genetic engineering from an industrialist's viewpoint, and discuss potential uses in areas such as agriculture, chemistry, mining and waste disposal.

The last three chapters of the book concentrate on the broader social issues of the new technology, and will, perhaps, be of the greatest general interest. If you are tempted to go straight to Chapters 9 and 10, no harm will be done, though it would be my hope that you would eventually return to find some snippets of interest in the earlier chapters.

2
The Organization of Life

Over three and a half billion years ago, when the conditions of temperature, chemical composition and radiant energy were just right, life appeared on earth. Most probably, this happened in the sea, and on a unique occasion. In other words, the wild profusion of living forms from the humblest of bacteria or algae to man himself, are all descended from the first primitive living cell. As we shall see, this carries profound implications for genetic engineering. In this chapter we shall describe the cell as the basic common element of all living matter, and will show how cells build up tissues, organs and eventually an individual. Looking deeply into the cell, we will come to grips with the intracellular structures and the molecules that make them up. This will bring us to the central role of DNA in the life process and the reasons why different cells in the body perform very different functions.

The Cell–a Fundamental Unit of Living Matter

One of the utopian dreams of science is to build up a continuum of knowledge about the universe that describes and explains nature in terms of its smallest building blocks. Subatomic particles make up atoms; atoms come together to build molecules; molecules aggregate, often in very complex ways, to build substances, objects, organisms and so forth. Objects and organisms form parts of collective wholes such as families, societies and civilizations. All the matter and life on earth constitutes a planet, which, however, is only part of a solar system in one galaxy of the universe. In practice, the limits of our understanding are such that, while we can make broad statements about how each component or level of complexity relates to the next higher level of organization, many important details remain obscure. In fact, there is a tendency for scientific enquiry to remain within the parameters of a particular level, gaining deeper and deeper insights into it, without worrying too much about connections to the level above or below. So nuclear physicists study subatomic particles; chemists, molecules; and geologists, rocks. While interfaces between disciplines sometimes bring forward the most exciting discoveries, most scientists choose not to venture beyond a given frame of reference.

An attempt to introduce biological phenomena to the layman runs into a similar problem: where to start? What level of organization is the most meaningful entry point to make the excitement of genetic engineering accessible? Most authors step right in and lead with a picture of the molecule, DNA. However, I have chosen to begin with a higher level of complexity, namely the cell, which, I have learnt, ought not to be taken for granted! When the cell and its parts have become familiar, the story of the molecules will be much easier to follow.

While there are significant differences between various sorts of cells, there are also sufficient similarities for it to be clear that the cell is the fundamental unit of living matter, or, in other words, that the first life form was a single-celled organism and that all subsequently evolved living species consist of a cell or cells. For convenience, Figure 1 represents an animal cell—plant cells or bacterial cells obey somewhat different rules. A typical animal cell is about one-thousandth of a centimetre (or one-two-and-a-half-thousandth of an inch) in diameter, which means that a single cell cannot be seen by the naked eye but can be easily recognized under even quite a simple microscope. The limits of the standard microscope are magnification factors of about a thousand, and if one needs to observe cells in still greater detail, a much more complex piece of equipment is required, the electron microscope. This instrument can magnify cells about 100 000-fold and has contributed notably to our present picture of cellular structure and organization. In a complex multicellular organism such as ourselves, it is important to remember that every part—the liver, the brain, the muscles—is made up of cells, conforming to a basic pattern, but differing in detail.

It is convenient to think of a cell as something like an industrial factory. The first fundamental division of the cell is into two components, the nucleus and cytoplasm. The nucleus is like the office of the factory. It is the control centre of the cell, the place where the fundamental decisions are made about just what kind of work that particular cell is going to do. The

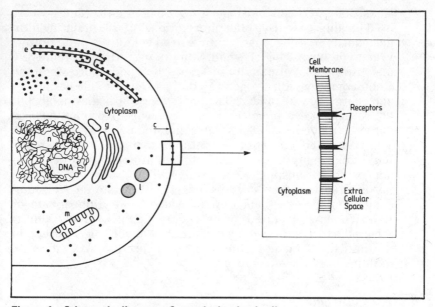

Figure 1 Schematic diagram of a typical animal cell
The most important organelles are shown: c, cell membrane; e, endoplasmic reticulum; g, Golgi apparatus; l, lysosomes; m, mitochondrion; n, nucleus; r, ribosome.

nucleus also contains the apparatus for self-replication of the cell by the process of division that we call mitosis. In contrast, the cytoplasm is the shop floor. It is the place where the work of the cell is done, where the machines and the assembly lines are efficiently positioned, and where the power is delivered where it is needed. The cytoplasm is not a random sea of molecules swimming around higgledy-piggledy, but rather a highly organized and compartmented structure. It contains parts which can be seen in the electron microscope and fished out and analysed by sophisticated biophysical and biochemical techniques. These parts are collectively referred to as subcellular organelles. Only the most important organelles are shown in figure 1.

Subcellular Organelles: the Mitochondria

The mitochondria are the powerhouses of the cell, creating little mobile packets of energy for use in the myriad chemical conversions that each cell must perform each minute. The process used is called oxidative phosphorylation, but this daunting term need not deter us because what we need to know is quite simple. When you burn a log of wood, you are performing a relatively uncontrolled act of oxidation. The carbon and hydrogen in the wood combine with oxygen to yield carbon dioxide gas, water and energy by way of heat. The energy is rapidly dissipated, but the mitochondria have figured out a way of promoting oxidation so that most of the energy generated is chemically stored. The controlled oxidation of cellular foodstuffs leads to the build-up of energy-rich, phosphate-containing molecules called adenosine triphosphate or simply ATP. Whenever the cell needs a bit of energy, it grabs a few of these stored ATP molecules and breaks them down to adenosine diphosphate or ADP. The energy stored in the energy-rich phosphate bond is released to drive the required chemical conversion, whereupon the hard-working mitochondria reconvert the ADP to ATP, building back the energy store.

The Lysosomes

The lysosomes are central to the digestive system of a cell. Cells take up a wide variety of substances from their environment. Some cells, such as the scavenger white cells of the blood, are big eaters and swallow particles such as invading microbes or bits of dead cells. Others take up only nutrient molcules present in the fluid around them. In either case, it is necessary to break down the material entering the cell into portions that can be used in cellular metabolism. This requires the action of digestive enzymes, and, as in the human stomach, an acid environment. If such enzymes and acids are spilt freely into the cytoplasm, the effects could be disastrous. Therefore, the cell keeps the enzymes and acids tucked away behind a barrier inside the lysosomes. The nutrients are at first also kept in little bags or pouches called vacuoles. The lysosomes discharge their contents into these food vacuoles so that digestion can proceed.

The Ribosomes

Scattered throughout all cells there are tiny punctate organelles called ribosomes. Frequently these appear in aggregates of ten or twenty and then they are referred to as polyribosomes. The ribosomes are central to our story, because they are instruments involved in our reading the genetic code making the proteins which end up doing most of the work of the cell. We shall discuss their function more fully when we meet messenger RNA.

The Endoplasmic Reticulum

When the cell makes proteins for its own internal use, the ribosomes concerned lie free inside the cytoplasm. However, many specialized cells make proteins which have to leave the cell and circulate in the blood to be of use to the body. A hormone like insulin is a typical example. Insulin is made by cells in the pancreas and regulates metabolic processes in virtually every cell of the body. Antibodies illustrate the point equally well. Antibodies are the proteins which recognize and neutralize foreign invaders that enter the body. They are made by a specialized cell type called a plasma cell, and are secreted by it, but may act anywhere that the bloodstream takes them. The endoplasmic reticulum is a kind of river system that guides the molecules destined for export to an appropriate packaging centre. The endoplasmic reticulum is made up of double membranes between which the protein molecules flow. The polyribosomes making proteins destined for export are actually attached to these membranes so that there can be no doubt about the newly synthesized export product getting to the right place.

The Golgi Apparatus

Proteins destined for secretion move to a system of membranes and sacs or pouches which sits in the cytoplasm right next to the nucleus. This is called the Golgi apparatus and is a concentrating and packaging centre. When the proteins are ready for export from the cell, they move in tiny bubbles from the Golgi to the surface of the cell, where they are released. At various points in the journey from endoplasmic reticulum to outside the cell, sugars may be linked on to the proteins, an important point for our later consideration, as genetically engineered bacteria fail to perform this function.

The Cell Membrane

Though not an organelle, the outer skin of the cell, the cell membrane, requires special comment. Chemical reactions inside the cell occur in a watery environment, and there is also a watery milieu outside the cell called the extracellular fluid. What separates the molecules inside the cell from the outside world is a skin largely made up of fats or lipids. This skin, the cell membrane, is impermeable to most molecules, thereby preserving the cell's autonomy and integrity. Obviously, therefore, when molecules need to get in, to feed the cell or deliver messages, or when molecules need to get out, say to provide the bloodstream with some secretion, special channelling devices of various sorts need to be created. The membrane is therefore a very dynamic and functional entity. Floating in the sea of fat we find a large number of proteins, and some of these function as sensitive antennae, constructed to receive signals and messages of various sorts from neighbouring cells or from hormones in the bathing fluid. These molecules are called cell membrane receptors.

The Macromolecules of Life

Living cells have plenty of small molecules in them, such as water, salts, sugars and organic chemicals that perform specialized tasks or act as building blocks. However, somehow it is the large molecules or macromolecules that are most characteristic of living matter. These come in four varieties, namely nucleic acids, proteins, carbohydrates and fats. Carbohydrates and fats in the main serve structural and energy-storage functions. Interesting though they are, they need not detain us at this point. The molecules that the budding student of genetic engineering must come to grips with are the nucleic acids and the proteins. Some proteins are also useful for their structural properties, such as the keratin which makes up hair, and we are less concerned with these than the so-called globular proteins which perform much more specialized and dynamic tasks in the body.

The Proteins

Proteins are really cunningly designed molecular machines which eons of evolution have painstakingly built to be superbly efficient at one task each. Nobody knows exactly how many different sorts of proteins exist in, for example, the human body, but in terms of order of magnitude, a hundred thousand is not a bad guess. Moreover, some proteins come as variations on a theme, the most extreme example being the antibodies protecting us against infectious diseases. These really represent only eight sorts of proteins, but tiny, subtle variations in structure make it possible for a person to manufacture a hundred million different antibodies each targeted against a different foreign invader. So it will be a very long time indeed till mankind knows the structure of all or even most of the proteins which an individual possesses. This is a pity, because it is in essence differences in proteins which determine differences in functional behaviour of cells, and therefore, eventually, of whole individuals.

The key workhorses of the cell are proteins called enzymes. An enzyme is a catalyst. It encourages a particular chemical reaction to proceed with speed and efficiency. Enzymes are therefore essential for most of the synthetic and degradative processes that go on in the body. Enzymes break down food, help in the transport and storage of energy, are vitally involved in the synthesis of all macromolecules, and obviously are crucial to the replication of the cell. The most important property of an enzyme is its *specificity*. The enzyme which breaks down ordinary sugar into its component parts does not act on sugar of milk, which has its own enzyme. Neither one can metabolize the larger storage carbohydrate, glycogen. The specificity of an enzyme depends on its having a particular topological region on its surface with a pattern that is complementary to a corresponding site on the molecule on which the enzyme acts, namely the *substrate*. This congruence of shapes encourages enzyme and substrate to stick to each other when they meet through random molecular motion. Attached to its substrate, the enzyme can do its work. Frequently, the reaction being catalysed actually depends on some different portion of the enzyme molecule than the initial combining site. Also, attachment to its substrate may cause a slight change in shape in the enzyme. A new active site may thus be exposed. Such a change in shape is known as an allosteric effect.

In many cases, a particular chemical conversion involves a series or cascade of sequential enzymic reactions. This may mean that a whole row of enzymes is arrayed in the correct spatial order on a specialized membrane framework. Each enzyme does one specific portion of a planned programme of work and it does so by behaving rather like a machine. So the analogy to an assembly line in a factory is very close.

Other proteins, which are not enzymes, also display the same great specificity. Antibodies, which neutralize poisons and microbes that enter the body, are specific: an anti-measles antibody has no effect against poliomyelitis. Haemoglobin has the specific capacity to take up oxygen in the lungs, where the concentration of oxygen is high, and to release it in the tissues, where the concentration is lower because the oxygen is being used up by the cells. Once again, haemoglobin does this single, vital job by undergoing appropriate changes in shape to snap up and then release the oxygen. So, clearly, the shape of proteins is central to their correct function. A highly sophisticated science called X-ray crystallography has revealed the detailed shape of many proteins down to the exact position of the constituent atoms in relation to one another. The technique can magnify proteins one hundred million times and it is quite fun to walk into an X-ray crystallographer's laboratory and literally walk around a model of a single protein molecule that occupies half a room. Often, the shape gives the clue to how the molecular machine works.

Amino Acids: the Building Blocks for Proteins

How does each protein get the special shape it needs to fulfil its mission in life? The answer to that lies in the arrangement of the individual building blocks that make up the protein. Like all the macromolecules, proteins are polymers made up of smaller component parts. These small molecules, weighing about one hundred times more than a hydrogen atom, are called amino acids. There are twenty different amino acids making up the proteins of living cells. They all have names, of course, but more importantly, each has its own characteristic shape. A typical protein will consist of fifty to two thousand amino acids, with the building blocks arranged in all manner of spatial configurations. You can imagine the vast number of different shapes which that master creator, evolution, has been able to fashion through different arrangements of the twenty different shaped bricks.

One deep truth about proteins must be appreciated before the genetic code can be understood. The individual amino acids are coupled together one at a time as a protein is synthesized. A single amino acid attaches to the ribosome to begin the process. Then enzymes couple on the next amino acid, then the next, and so on, one by one, till the full chain of amino acids is complete. One can therefore describe a protein as a linear array of amino acids, one after another. This description, however, neglects the fact that the linear array really folds up into a complex, three-dimensional shape. Therefore, as the molecule assumes its final form, amino acid number 3 may find itself just as close, in space, to amino acid 32 or 51 as it is to its neighbours, amino acids numbers 2 and 4. Nevertheless, the final shape of the protein under the conditions of the cellular milieu is an obligate consequence of the sequence of amino acids, the *primary structure*, as it is called. The folding follows from the pushes and pulls that the sequential elements of the chain exert on one another. So, in the end, if evolution wishes to tinker with a particular protein, all it has to ensure is a change in order, and a subtle change in final shape will assuredly follow.

The names of the twenty amino acids will not concern us much for the purposes of this book. We shall meet them shortly when considering the genetic code. When protein chemists analyse the sequence of proteins, they frequently make use of one of two conventions when writing up their results. Rather than reporting the structure as a series of full names, they will designate each amino acid by its first three letters, or by a single, arbitrarily chosen letter of the alphabet.

The Nucleic Acids

The other biopolymers or macromolecules of deep concern to us are the nucleic acids. These, too, are composed of building blocks called nucleotides. The nucleotides are a little more complicated than the amino acids, because each consists of a base, a sugar and a phosphate group. This complexity need not bother us, however, because the sugar-phosphate portion really serves only a structural function. The information content, or coding function, is all tied up with the bases. And now we come to the crucial conceptual difference between the proteins and the nucleic acids. The function of the proteins depends on their final three-dimensional shape. They are machines, working objects. The function of the nucleic acids depends only on the linear order of the bases. They are blueprints or code-books— useful only when translated.

There are two sorts of nucleic acids, DNA and RNA, or deoxyribonucleic acid and ribonucleic acid, to dignify them with their full names. The key point about DNA is that it is a string of genes, and each gene contains the coded information for one protein. The DNA is responsible for the master architectural blueprint, held permanently in the head office, the nucleus. RNA comes in various types, but the most important from our point of view, the messenger RNA, is more like a shop drawing—a modified copy of the DNA which actually moves from nucleus to cytoplasm, and is used there, on the shop floor, where the proteins are made. Both DNA and RNA use only four bases each to perform their coding function. The bases of DNA consist of two molecules with a double organic ring structure, adenine and guanine, and two with just a single ring structure, cytosine and thymine. It is a fortunate thing for the sanity of molecular biologists that these four names begin with different letters of the alphabet; they can conveniently be referred to as just A, G, C and T. RNA also uses A, G and C, but instead of T it uses the chemically rather similar base uracil or U, which, in coding terms, is equivalent to T.

The DNA in the nucleus exists as paired strands of circular staircase-like assemblies—the famous double helix of James Watson and Francis Crick (Figure 2). The repeats of sugar and phosphate form the backbones of the strands, and the bases, A, G, C and T, poke in towards the middle. In fact, the bases of the two strands pair up through a particular type of chemical bond called hydrogen bonding. A always pairs up with T and G with C. When it is time for a cell to divide, which obviously requires the whole genetic machinery of the cell to be faithfully copied, the double helix unwinds and enzymes create a new strand complementary to the old one, inserting a T opposite an A, a C opposite a G, an A opposite a T, a G opposite a C and so forth. A simple bacterial cell has just over three million such base pairs in its total DNA, already representing an enormous coding potential. This DNA exists as a single large double-helical molecule. A human cell contains a thousand-fold more DNA again! Presumably to facilitate the organization of all this genetic material, the DNA of human cells is broken into forty-six separate chunks called chromosomes. Of these, forty-four come as identical pairs, and two are the sex chromosomes, X and X in the female and X and Y in the male. Each chromosome contains a single very long molecule of double-helical DNA, and it also contains some proteins called histones which are tightly bound to the DNA and which may have some regulatory function.

The Genetic Code

We come now to a concept which confuses many people, but which, essentially, is quite simple. It is that of the genetic code. Consider for a moment the universe of our daily lives. It is filled with objects and entities—buildings, streets, cars, furniture, people, animals. We want to communicate with each other about all these objects and the processes through which they are related. This is the function of language, and moreover we have learnt to record that language in written form. We can

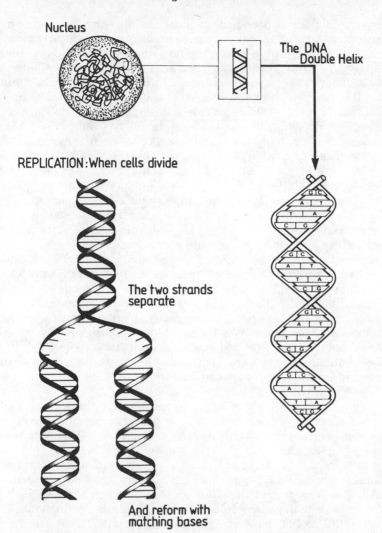

Nucleus

The DNA Double Helix

REPLICATION: When cells divide

The two strands separate

And reform with matching bases

Figure 2 The DNA double helix
The backbone of each helical strand consists of repeating sugar and phosphate units. The coding function is carried out by 4 bases, adenine, thymine, guanine and cytosine (A, T, G and C). In double-stranded DNA, the bases are always paired and bonded together in the middle of the helix, A always pairing with T and G with C. When DNA replicates itself prior to cell division, the two strands of the double helix separate and each strand serves as the template for the construction of a second, complementary strand. Enzymes ensure that, wherever the parent strand to be replicated possesses an A, the incoming building block will be a T, and so forth.

regard English as a code that has the following features. The simplest element of the code is a letter, one of twenty-six possible choices in the alphabet. The letters are strung together linearly to form words, most of which are two to fifteen letters long. The words when read by the human eye and brain stand for the real objects and processes that we are trying to describe. In a sense, they gain their reality through the translation process. So it is with the genetic code. Instead of English, with its twenty-six letter alphabet, which, packaged into words, has given us all of Shakespeare and also over a hundred volumes of the *Journal of Immunology*, the genetic code has only four letters in its alphabet, A, G, C and T (or its equivalent U). The linear sequence of these four letters in the DNA of each species contains the information for a bee or a sunflower or an elephant or an Albert Einstein. Just as in English, there is a need for punctuation and notations to indicate where words or sentences start and stop. And just as in English, the coded message of the gene gains its reality only when translated in the form of a protein. So the essence of the genetic code is how DNA codes for proteins. Essentially (though there are important exceptions) one gene codes for one protein. This raises the question of how the language of the genes, with its four-letter alphabet, can be translated into the language of proteins with its twenty-letter alphabet. Actually, a cryptographer could come up with a number of elegant solutions to that problem, but nature has found just one, which is universal to each living species.

First of all, the code is linear or sequential. The sequence of bases specifies the sequence of amino acids. Secondly, the code is non-overlapping—that is, a gene segment AGCTGTA cannot be read either as AGC, TGT, A. . or as . .A, GCT, GTA. Thirdly, it is a triplet code. A sequence of three bases codes for one amino acid, thus AGC codes for an amino acid called serine, while ACG signifies the amino acid threonine, and so forth. Such base triplets are called codons, and, given the 4 bases, there are 4x4x4 or sixty-four codons in all. There are only twenty amino acids to code for, so we have coding information to spare. Three of the codons are used as 'stop' signs, i.e. are punctuation marks. Spare information is obviously available, so most amino acids can, in fact, be coded for by more than one triplet. It turns out that, frequently, the first two letters of the codon are the key ones, and the third does not matter very much. This point is illustrated when we look at a Table which spells out the genetic code in total. There is, of course, no need to remember the details, but here is how the genetic code looks.

The genetic code

Codon	Amino Acid	Codon	Amino Acid	Codon	Amino Acid	Codon	Amino Acid
UUU	Phenylalanine	CUU	Leucine	AUU	Isoleucine	GUU	Valine
UUC	Phenylalanine	CUC	Leucine	AUC	Isoleucine	GUC	Valine
UUA	Leucine	CUA	Leucine	AUA	Isoleucine	GUA	Valine
UUG	Leucine	CUG	Leucine	AUG	Methionine	GUG	Valine
UCU	Serine	CCU	Proline	ACU	Threonine	GCU	Alanine
UCC	Serine	CCC	Proline	ACC	Threonine	GCC	Alanine
UCA	Serine	CCA	Proline	ACA	Threonine	GCA	Alanine
UCG	Serine	CCG	Proline	ACG	Threonine	GCG	Alanine
UAU	Tyrosine	CAU	Histidine	AAU	Asparagine	GAU	Aspartic acid
UAC	Tyrosine	CAC	Histidine	AAC	Asparagine	GAC	Aspartic acid
UAA	STOP	CAA	Glutamine	AAA	Lysine	GAA	Glutamic acid
UAG	STOP	CAG	Glutamine	AAG	Lysine	GAG	Glutamic acid
UGU	Cysteine	CGU	Arginine	AGU	Serine	GGU	Glycine
UGC	Cysteine	CGC	Arginine	AGC	Serine	GGC	Glycine
UGA	STOP	CGA	Arginine	AGA	Arginine	GGA	Glycine
UGG	Tryptophan	CGG	Arginine	AGG	Arginine	GGG	Glycine

The four bases of RNA are used—remember U is equivalent to T.

Reading the Genetic Code

Given these basic elements of the code, how do the events of protein synthesis actually unfold? Messages coming from inside or outside a cell tell the DNA of the genes that it is time for a particular protein to be made. This process of *gene activation* can be likened to turning on an electric light switch. The capacity for all that light was there all along, but only when the switch is turned is the capacity actualized. When a gene is activated (remember: one gene, one protein), the events depicted in Figure 3 unfold. First, an acurate copy of the DNA's genetic message is made in RNA. The DNA acts as a template, and the RNA copy of the gene, still at this moment within the nucleus of the cell, is called a *primary transcript*. The process of copying DNA information into RNA information is referred to as transcription. For reasons that are, as yet, by no means clear, the coding information of a gene in cells of higher organisms, including humans, is often interrupted by stretches of bases that have no coding function. These 'nonsense' stretches are referred to as intervening sequences or introns, and the portions with coding information are exons. The primary RNA transcript is a faithful copy of both exons and introns. Before moving to the cytoplasm, the primary transcript is processed so that the bits corresponding to introns are snipped out of the RNA strand, and it is sealed up to reflect accurately the exons only. The RNA is now ready to move to the cytoplasm as *messenger RNA*.

Within the cytoplasm, ribosomes attach themselves to the messenger RNA strand and the process of copying the coded information into an amino acid sequence begins. This is called *translation*. You can think of ribosomes as being akin to the head of a magnetic tape machine which reads the messages on the tape as it moves along. In fact, it is a little more complicated than that, because the codons are actually read by *anticodons*, RNA triplets on an adaptor molecule called transfer RNA, there being specific transfer RNAs for each amino acid. These transfer RNAs ferry the right amino acid along to the ribosome, and appropriate enzymes link each one to the growing protein chain. As the ribosome moves along to the next codon on the messenger RNA, a new transfer RNA brings up the new amino acid, and so forth. Ribosomes travel along messenger RNA at a set rate. For efficiency, as many as possible will attach themselves, evenly spaced about 100 bases apart, to one RNA molecule, which thereby is read simultaneously by several ribosomes. The longer the message, the more ribosomes crowd on. The size of a polyribosome is therefore a reflection of the size of the protein being made.

When the protein chain in completed, it falls off the ribosome and finds itself either free in the cytoplasm or inside the endoplasmic reticulum. It folds and coils into the shape already inherent in the amino acid sequence. In some cases, specific enzymes attach sugar molecules to the protein. Furthermore, many important proteins are actually mixtures of several differ-

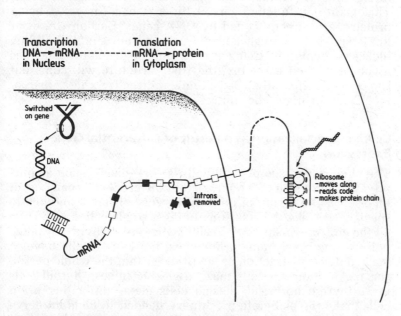

Figure 3   Sequential events in gene activation
When a gene is activated, the two strands of the DNA double helix separate, and a messenger RNA copy of one of the strands is made. This step is termed transcription. In animal cells, the gene contains stretches of DNA with coding function, called exons, and intervening sections of DNA which do not code for protein and the function of which is unknown. These are called introns. As the primary RNA transcript is a faithful copy of DNA, it also contains sequences corresponding to exons and to introns. Inside the nucleus, the messenger RNA is processed so that the intron sequences are cut out and the cuts are sealed up. This processed messenger RNA then moves to the cytoplasm. Here, ribosomes attach to the messenger RNA and a protein chain is progressively assembled, each triplet of three bases coding for one particular amino acid. When the ribosome comes to the end of the messenger RNA, it falls off and the completed protein is released.

ent proteins, and in that case the component proteins are often referred to as *chains*. For example, the insulin molecule consists of one chain of twenty-one amino acids linked to a second chain of thirty amino acids. Antibody molecules consist of four chains, two identical light chains of about 220 amino acids each, and two identical heavy chains which are over twice as long. Clearly, if a protein is to be made by genetic engineering, the need to make more than one chain and hook them together correctly will make the task a little harder.

We have not yet said how the genetic code dictates the structure of other macromolecules, such as carbohydrates or lipids. This again is a function served by enzymes. Enzymes, being proteins, are directly coded by DNA genes. Carbohydrates or lipids are built through enzyme action from simple building blocks. If evolution changes even one of the many enzymes involved in their assembly, the final structure will come out somewhat differently. So, albeit indirectly, these macromolecules are under the control of the genes as well.

Cellular Specialization as a Result of Differential Gene Expression

The chief advantage of multicellular organisms, such as ourselves, is a division of labour, so that different cells can permit themselves the luxury of performing very different and highly specialized tasks. A bacterium, being a single cell, has to have all the enzymic machinery to eat, swim, grow, divide, produce poisons, etc. In a human, however, individual cells have to make only a tiny fraction of the proteins that the whole person can make. Stomach cells make digestive juices; thyroid cells make thyroid hormone; plasma cells make antibodies; brain cells make the elaborate machinery needed to conduct nerve impulses. Clearly, then, only a small proportion of the total person's genes are activated in one particular cell. Presumably, nature could have used one of two strategies to achieve this end. It could have decreed that cells on the way to becoming specialized discarded the genes they did not need. However, this would have allowed little flexibility. A cell could never 'change its mind' about its function. Alternatively, each cell could retain all the genes of the whole organism. The assumption of specialized function would then represent a turning on of certain genes and a turning off of the majority. This second strategy is the one that nature in fact adopted. It means that cellular specialization is the result of differential activation of sets of genes in different cells. The study of gene activation as a key to the process of the formation of specialized organs and tissues is one of the most fascinating and rapidly moving areas of modern cell biology. When it is a little more advanced, it will tell us not only how a liver came to be a liver, a heart a heart and so forth; it will also tell us a great deal more about how they differ, and thus, how they function.

Nature has its own 'plans', its own way of doing things, but man is the wild card in the pack. Before we turn to a consideration of how he learnt to trick the genes, let us reiterate what is important for later chapters. Each cell contains the genes of the whole individual, as very long strands of double-helical DNA molecules. The DNA, composed of a linear array of four basic coding units, is copied or transcribed into RNA when a gene is activated. After some processing, this RNA is transported from the nucleus of the cell into its cytoplasm, and there acts as template for the building of proteins. A triplet code ensures that the instructions given in the four-letter alphabet of the DNA and RNA are faithfully translated into the twenty-letter alphabet of the proteins. One gene codes for one protein, and different cells activate different genes, so making different sets of proteins. Therefore each cell is fitted for different tasks.

3

The Mechanics of Gene Transplantation

Now that we have a reasonable working knowledge of the molecular organization of life, we may ask why anyone would wish to tinker with such a perfect machinery? DNA encodes the information for life, RNA copies allow this to be translated into beautiful and useful proteins—who needs more? The answer, as usual in science, revolves around the twin thirsts, for knowledge and power. To know more about the genes, we need techniques that can give us a gene in pure form and in sufficient amount for detailed chemical analysis. To harness this knowledge for socially useful purposes, we need methods to transplant the gene to rapidly-growing organisms, and to switch it on, as desired, for the mass production of precious proteins. Within a brief decade an engineering technology of peerless elegance and amazing sophistication has been developed which allows all this and more. Biology will never be the same again.

The trouble with the DNA in a cell is that you cannot see the wood for the trees. The molecules are so long and contain thousands of genes. The opening gambit of the genetic engineer is to break the DNA up into small, manageable bits, each containing one or just a few genes. Each little bit, one at a time, is stitched into a special, virus-like piece of DNA gifted with the ability for self-replication. These virus-like, recombined DNA molecules now invade rapidly-dividing host cells, again one at a time. Each host cell, frequently a bacterium or a yeast, thereby becomes a factory for one pure gene. Clever tricks allow the genetic engineer to pick out the host cell carrying the gene wanted for that particular experiment. By isolating that one special cell, and growing it up to any desired quantity, the one desired gene (or its protein product) can be obtained. So four basic steps are common to all of genetic engineering. First, break the DNA up into short stretches. Secondly, anneal each bit to a suitable ferryman. Thirdly, have these ferrymen invade host cells one at a time, and grow up large numbers. Finally, find the cells with the right transplanted genes in them.

In this chapter we shall uncover the 'nuts and bolts' of genetic engineering technology, describing the key tools and procedures. This will allow us to look at some of the fascinating practical uses in later chapters without pausing too long to worry about methods. If you find the rest of this chapter too technical, skip straight to the summary at the end. Do not think of this as a defeat; even pared down to its bare bones, the engineering is hard to follow in detail, and it would be a pity to miss the other messages of this book through frustration over Chapter 3!

Restriction Endonucleases: Precision Tools Par Excellence

Consider the human genes: a total of three thousand million base pairs broken up into the chromosomes, each chromosomal double helix still being scores of millions of base pairs long. How to find a given gene? How to study its structure, when there is only a single copy per cell? How to separate it out from all the other DNA, prior to transplanting it? The genetic engineer needs precision tools *par excellence* for these endeavours, and the beginning point is a series of enzymes called restriction endonucleases.

The restriction endonucleases are enzymes that cut the DNA double helix in very precise ways. They have the capacity to recognize specific base sequences on DNA and then to cut each strand at a given place. For example, the frequently used enzyme EcoRI recognizes the portion of the double helix reading:

$$-G-A-A-T-T-C-$$
$$-C-T-T-A-A-G-$$

It makes a very precise cut between the G and the A in each strand leaving the DNA looking like this:

$$-G$$
$$-C-T-T-A-A$$

and

$$A-A-T-T-C-$$
$$G-$$

Obviously, the enzyme will cut a very long DNA double helix many times, in fact every time the particular series of bases turns up in the code. This creates a mixture of fragments of DNA (known as a DNA digest), still in double-helical form, but with a short stretch of single-stranded DNA poking out at both ends of each fragment. These short strands are often termed 'sticky ends'. One of the basic features of DNA is that, under suitable chemical conditions, bases 'want to' pair up with each other, A to T, G to C, T to A, C to G. If this is so for a single base pair, it is all the more 'intense a desire' for complementary stretches, so −T−T−A−A very much 'wants to' pair up with A−A−T−T−. Having made the set of cuts with the restriction enzyme, the scientist can set up conditions where the fragments now meet up again, sticky end pairing with its complementary partner. The DNA cuts can be repaired by separate special enzymes called DNA ligases. In the process, of course, it will only occasionally happen that a particular fragment pairs up with the fragment that was its previous neighbour. The likelihood is that, in the mixture of thousands of fragments, a quite random and new arrangement of DNA will result. That is the first basic clue to genetic engineering.

Not all restriction endonucleases leave sticky ends. Consider the enzyme Hpa I. It recognizes stretches of the double helix reading

$$-G-T-T-A-A-C-$$
$$-C-A-A-T-T-G-$$

and in fact cuts the two strands right through the middle of the sequence, between the T and the A of one strand, the A and the T of the second. This leaves fragments with flush ends, with no spontaneous desire to recombine. However, this is no desperate problem for the recombinant DNA technologist wishing to use this enzyme. He simply puts a 'tail' of −T−T−T−T−T on to the end of one strand of some fragments, and of A−A−A−A−A− on to one strand of others, thereby creating the desired sticky ends through organic chemistry. The trick is known as *homopolymer tailing*. Furthermore, not all restriction endonucleases require six base pairs to be lined up in a special sequence. For instance, the enzyme Hha I recognizes the sequence

$$-G-C-G-C-$$
$$-C-G-C-G-$$

and cuts each strand where shown by the dashed line, thus:

$$-G-C-G \dashv C-$$
$$-C \vdash G-C-G-$$

The three examples of restriction enzymes illustrate one common point about the sites on the DNA double helix being recognized. In each case, and indeed for the whole family of these enzymes, the stretch of base pairs recognized reads the same forwards as backwards. The word palindrome describes a word (like radar), or a phrase (Madam I'm Adam) that reads the same from left to right as from right to left. All the sites able to be recognized by restriction endonucleases possess *palindromic* sequences. This symmetry appears to be essential for the enzyme to act to break the DNA double helix. There are now about three hundred restriction endonucleases to choose from, giving the genetic engineer a whole battery of precision instruments. Before we come to what use the genetic engineer makes of these enzymes, we should ask why nature bothered to invent them. In the bacterial world, the enzymes seem to be a protection against foreign DNA which might enter a bacterium and interfere with its function. The bacterium's own DNA is not degraded by its own endonucleases, because it pops a little protective molecule (a methyl group, in fact) on to the recognition site for its own restriction enzymes. This blocks cleavage, but the restriction enzyme is free to attack other non-methylated DNA that enters, provided always that this possesses the right sequence of bases somewhere along its length.

Restriction Endonucleases in Genetic Engineering

The prime use of restriction endonucleases is to break the long DNA double helix into smaller, more manageable bits. Suppose you wished to study an automobile to find out how it functioned. This would be rather difficult if you could not take it to pieces. But by judiciously sorting out the components (gear box, differential, distributor, engine head and so on) and attacking each as an organizational entity, we render the problem more accessible. So it is with DNA. The genetic engineer, beginning to study the structure of a particular gene of interest, does not know where a site for a particular endonuclease might lie. But in trying the various enzymes anyway, the parent DNA molecule is broken into specific fragments that are more readily analysed and manipulated.

Obviously, the longer the stretch of double helix acting as the recognized sequence for a restriction enzyme, the more rarely will it occur, and therefore the bigger the bits of DNA prepared by that particular enzyme. Most of the enzymes recognize stretches of four to six base pairs. If the bases were aligned at random in a stretch a million bases long, a particular sequence of four, say –G–C–G–C–, will occur *on average* once for every 4x4x4x4 or 256 bases. However, just as in tossing a coin, where on average 'heads' occurs half the time and 'tails' half the time, but strange runs of six heads in a row are not infrequent, it is perfectly possible to find a stretch of fifty bases where —G—C—G—C— turns up twice, or one of a thousand bases where it does not turn up at all. So the pieces of DNA prepared by the relevant enzyme Hha I, while *averaging* 256 base pairs in length, are in fact very heterogeneous in length. If the genetic engineer allows the enzyme to act for a long time, until every last recognition site has been attacked by the enzyme, the million-long molecule of DNA should yield slightly fewer than four thousand different pieces. In practice, it is frequently convenient to allow the restriction endonuclease to act for a suboptimal length of time, resulting in some —G—C—G—C— stretches *not* being cleaved. Then random chance will ensure that, if you start not with one DNA molecule but with a large number, particular —G—C—G—C— stretches, say forming part of the gene you are interested in, will escape breakage. The heterogeneity in fragmentation is increased by this manoeuvre. A restriction endonuclease recognizing six base stretches, such as EcoRI, will find a suitable area for attack only once every 4096 base pairs. Again, for incomplete enzymic digestion, the above rules apply. So the genetic engineer can break up DNA in all sorts of ways, and learns by experience which enzymes are best for particular purposes. The principle is simply illustrated in Figure 4.

Having created this heterogeneous mixture of shorter stretches of DNA, the scientist can separate pieces on the basis of their size by well-established methods. For example, one can use a kind of molecular sieving technique known as gel electrophoresis. For DNA pieces consisting of fewer than a thousand base pairs, scientists use gels made of polyacrylamide. For larger molecules, up to many thousands of base pairs, more porous gels composed of agarose are used. In this way, scientists can get a kind of fingerprint of a DNA digest. If a fraction of interest is isolated, it can then be attacked by a second restriction enzyme, and if there is a site for that enzyme, a still smaller bit of DNA results. A map of restriction endonuclease sites on a stretch of DNA is a very useful first step in an analysis of its structure.

Vectors for the Cloning of DNA in Bacteria

We mentioned that the second step after breaking DNA was to stitch each piece into a self-replicating, virus-like stretch of DNA with the capacity to invade certain host cells. As a class, these useful ferrymen for the gene transplanter are known as vectors, and we must learn a little about them. Vectors are

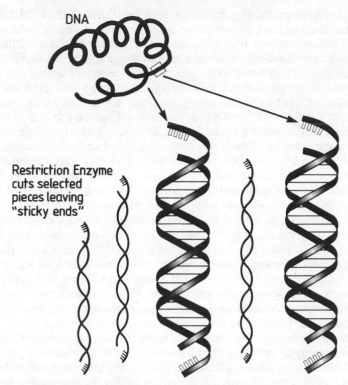

Figure 4 The first step in genetic engineering
DNA to be engineered is broken into small pieces. Restriction endonuclease enzymes recognize a particular sequence and cut the DNA double helix only where such a sequence appears. The resultant shorter stretches of DNA often have 'sticky ends'.

any genetic element that can carry genes about for the genetic engineer.

Bacteria are primitive organisms consisting of just one cell. In the popular mind, bacteria are thought of as harmful, disease-causing microbes. In fact, there are thousands of species of harmless bacteria occupying particular ecological niches in the biosphere. Many of these are useful, helping to produce vitamins in our intestines, co-operating with plants to allow them to use atmospheric nitrogen as a building block, or fermenting milk into cheese. Bacteria typically have one large circular double-stranded DNA molecule controlling their life and reproduction. As mentioned before, this is about three million base pairs long. Many bacteria also contain smaller double-stranded circular DNA molecules called *plasmids*. These are anywhere from two thousand to a few hundred thousand base pairs long. Plasmids have various curious properties. First, the genes they carry may not be absolutely essential for life and so a plasmid can sometimes leave one bacterial cell and enter another, thereby transferring genetic traits between cells. Secondly, the plasmid can reproduce itself inside the bacterium independently of the main bacterial DNA. Thirdly, a plasmid can sometimes fuse with the main DNA and later work its way loose again, but in such a manner as to drag a piece of the main DNA with it. Nature seems to have evolved plasmids as an efficient way of exchanging genes between bacterial cells. Plasmids are one vital family of vectors for the genetic engineer.

Surprisingly, bacteria also sometimes catch a virus! Viruses are the very smallest forms of life, and they are true parasites, being able to live only inside a cell. Bacterial viruses are called *phages* as they sometimes 'eat' the bacterium, at least in the sense of killing it and making it burst. The DNA of a typical phage would be fifty thousand bases long. The virus moves freely from bacterium to bacterium—in fact it possesses a very precise and beautifully designed mechanism for pricking the bacterial wall and injecting its DNA. Phages, also, can sometimes integrate into the main bacterial DNA. When that happens, the virus stops annoying the host bacterium and lies quietly there, replicating only when the bacterium as a whole replicates. Over the years, scientists have worked out tricks to make phages jump into and out of the main DNA chromosome whenever they want. When the phage jumps out, it sometimes carries a host gene or two out with it. Phages are a second family of vectors.

So, these two sorts of self-replicating entities, plasmids and phages, have become key tools for the genetic engineer. Perhaps you have guessed the trick used for the second step in genetic engineering. A population of phages or plasmids is split open by a restriction endonuclease. Pieces of foreign DNA, with appropriate 'sticky ends' prepared through action of the same endonuclease, are added. Frequently, a foreign gene joins up with the plasmid or phage and, with appropriate enzymes, the circle is resealed. Hey presto, you have recombinant DNA! The plasmid or phage is allowed to infect bacteria and so acts as a vector for the foreign gene. Both vector and bacterial host divide as many times as the investigator wishes, and the foreign gene merrily divides with them. Bearing in mind that a bacterium can divide into two every twenty minutes, a billion-fold increase in the foreign DNA can be achieved in ten hours. A variety of vectors now exists, tailor-made for genetic engineering, some of them capable of transporting DNA fragments as long as forty thousand bases. There are even vectors called cosmids which combine the best features of phages and plasmids. Placing a vector with a particular, single gene in it into a bacterial cell and then growing billions of progeny is known as *cloning* that gene. A clone is just a technical term for a population descended from a single ancestor by non-sexual means. Cloning genes is not to be confused with the spectacular technique whereby amphibia such as tadpoles can be produced as identical sets by transplanting the nuclei of cells from one frog into a large number of frogs' eggs that have had their own nucleus removed. Cloning people, in that sense, is total science fiction. Cloning people's genes, as we shall see, is very much a daily reality.

Creating a Gene Library

Let us now see how the cloning of, for example, the genes of a mouse actually takes place. Mouse tissue is minced up and the DNA is chemically purified by techniques that have been known for decades. The DNA is treated by a suitable restriction enzyme, for example, one that potentially produces bits of DNA with an average of 4096 base pairs. If the enzyme acts for a relatively short time, so that it can cut say only one-fifth of the relevant sites, the DNA fragments will, on average, be twenty thousand base pairs long. A suitable vector, say phage virus DNA, is also treated with the same endonuclease, say one producing sticky ends. The two are mixed and then treated with a suitable DNA ligase, a sealing enzyme that heals the cuts. The sticking together and sealing will be an entirely random affair. Sometimes the sticky ends of the phage just join up with each other, re-forming the original, unaltered vector. In other cases, a random bit of the mouse DNA will join up with the two sticky ends of the vector, and the circle reseals with a bit of mouse DNA inserted into the vector to yield recombinant DNA. As the sextuplet of base pairs recognized by the restriction enzyme in our example will not occur regularly and exactly each 4096 base pairs, there will be bits of DNA of various sizes going in, the upper limit being defined by just what each particular vector can accommodate, forty thousand base pairs being the present maximum. Figure 5 shows the principle involved.

The scientist is now ready for step 3 of genetic engineering, namely to insert the vectors into host bacteria one at a time. First, by sophisticated, elegant methods, one must package the vector DNA in a surrounding coating that helps penetration of target bacteria. Then the genetically engineered vectors are mixed with a population of bacteria that has been grown in a soup-like nutrient broth. A proportion of the bacteria becomes infected, but at first the scientist does not know which ones. A

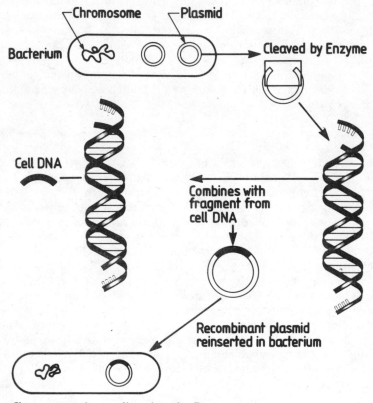

Figure 5 The second step in genetic engineering
DNA is inserted into a vector. In the case shown, the vector is a bacterial plasmid. The plasmid is cleaved by the same restriction endonuclease as used for the DNA to be transplanted, leaving sticky ends complementary to those of that DNA. Bits of DNA pair up and frequently create a recombined plasmid. DNA cuts are repaired by suitable enzymes.

useful trick sometimes employed is to ensure that the vector, e.g. a plasmid, carries a gene which confers resistance to a particular antibiotic. Then, in the phase of bacterial growth following the entry of the plasmid, that antibiotic is added to the culture medium, so only bacteria that have taken up the vector (and therefore the resistance gene) can grow. Once infection of bacteria by the vectors has occurred, it is convenient to grow the bacteria not in a soup but on the surface of a jelly. This prevents individual bacteria from swimming around, and allows each bacterium to grow into a *colony* of millions of cells. Colonies are readily visible to the naked eye. Each colony carries a huge number of copies of the vector, and of such foreign DNA as may have been incorporated into it. The general principles are seen in Figure 6.

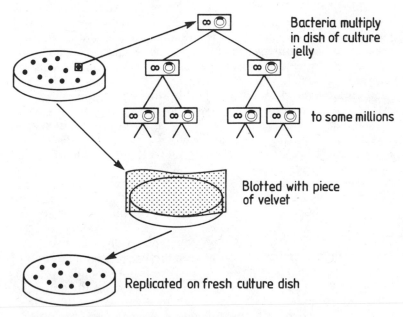

Figure 6   The third step in genetic engineering
Growth of bacteria carrying recombinant DNA: the plasmids are mixed with host E. coli bacteria, and the bacteria carrying recombinant plasmids are grown on the surface of a jellified culture medium. Each bacterium divides until a colony of some millions of bacteria is visible to the naked eye as a spot several millimetres in diameter. By carefully blotting the geographical pattern of colonies on to fresh jellified medium on a second culture dish, using a piece of velvet, a replica of the original dish can be made. As many replicas as desired can be produced.

A variant on this general theme is employed with phage vectors. As multiplying phages eventually destroy the bacteria in which they live, and infect neighbouring bacteria and destroy them also, one bacterium carrying a phage (in our case, a phage carrying a piece of foreign DNA) can make a hole in a lawn of growing bacteria. These holes are called plaques, and can again be spotted with the naked eye.

Let us now do a few simple calculations. In the example we have chosen, the average DNA insert will be twenty thousand pairs long. But the totality of the mouse's DNA, the mouse genome, as it is called, is over three thousand million base pairs. So 150 000 bacterial colonies (or phage plaques) will have within them approximately the total amount of DNA that was in the original mouse genome. Again random chance must be considered. It is quite possible that the 150 000 bacteria received a given stretch of DNA five times over, but that not even one bacterium received another stretch. So, to make reasonably sure that the total genome has somehow found its way into at least one bacterium, genetic engineers will usually prefer to use about ten times more altered bacteria, say 1.5 million in our example, to create the gene collection. Then a given gene will turn up, on average, ten times within the population, and virtually every gene should be present at least once. Moreover, as we have made only a partial DNA digest, even genes which have a restriction site in their middle will be present in the library because we have stopped the enzyme well before it has chewed up all the ten copies of the gene. Such a collection of bacteria or phage plaques is known as a *gene library*. Somewhere within the library, you will find the gene you want. Just as with an ordinary public library of books, the trick is to find what you want!

What we have just described is a library of *genomic* DNA. There are many occasions when the genetic engineer wants not a genomic library but one reflecting the information content of the messenger RNA of a particular population of cells. Remember, in any one cell type, only a small minority of the genes are active at any one time. Active genes are transcribed into RNA, which is processed in the nucleus and shipped out into the cytoplasm to initiate protein synthesis (Chapter 2). A particular cell's total messenger RNA therefore represents a small subset of the information content of genomic DNA. Moreover, the annoying little stretches of non-coding DNA, the introns, have been cut out during processing of the primary transcript. Suppose you are interested in a particular gene, say the one coding for haemoglobin. It makes good sense to get hold of some cells actively synthesizing haemoglobin, and to purify the messenger RNA from them. If you want to introduce a sophisticated trick, you can even purify the messenger RNA to yield molecules of just the right length to code for a haemoglobin chain. Then that population of RNA molecules can be copied into DNA by an enzyme called *reverse transcriptase*. This copy DNA, or cDNA for short, can be cloned into bacterial populations just as described for genomic DNA. A very much smaller library is now sure to have the information you want. You can get even more tricky than that. There are ways of getting rid of bits of cDNA that are common to two sorts of cells, and to purify that of one cell only—a good way of enriching for a specialized cDNA.

Screening the Library: How to find the Right Gene

The genetic engineer is now ready for Step 4. It is certainly clever to have ways of splitting DNA up into bits, and to produce vast amounts of each bit in colonies of bacteria. But how does one find the gene that you want? This is very much a needle in the haystack exercise. In the genomic library, only a few colonies, ten or fewer, amongst our collection of 1.5 million will have the gene we want. As we have seen, the situation is much better for a cDNA library. In devising the screening procedures, the genetic engineers have demonstrated both their genius and their industriousness.

We have already mentioned one clever trick, namely the gene for resistance to an antibiotic which is present in the vector. There is an elaboration of this principle which allows the discrimination of bacteria that have received a *recombinant* vector from ones that have received just an unaltered vector. The total population is grown in the presence of antibiotic 1, so getting only those bacteria carrying vectors. This transformed population is plated on a jelly dish, and colonies are grown up. There are now ways of making replicas of the geographical pattern of these growing colonies on jellified media containing all sorts of selective agents. Suppose the vector concerned carried a second resistance gene for antibiotic 2, and suppose further that a restriction endonuclease is chosen to 'open up' the plasmid or phage right in the middle of this second resistance gene. This time the enzyme is allowed to act for long enough to affect every plasmid. Obviously, then, if the vector's circular DNA rejoined intact, without a foreign DNA insert, the resistance gene would reseal, and the bacterium would grow in the presence of antibiotic 2. If, on the other hand, a bit of foreign DNA got attached and incorporated, the resistance gene would thereby have been interrupted and effectively destroyed. The bacterium which has received a vector with a DNA insert therefore cannot resist antibiotic 2, and fails to grow in it. The scientist then picks only those colonies on the original master plate that have *failed* to grow on the replica. There are many other ingenious ways to find only bacteria with recombinant DNA in them.

This is the relatively easy part. But what about finding bacteria that have not just any bit of foreign DNA, but the very one you want? We shall consider just two approaches to this, but bear in mind that there are many more. The first involves the 'desire' of complementary DNA strands to bind tightly to each other. Suppose you know the amino acid sequence of the protein for which you are seeking the gene, or even know just one short stretch of sequence data five amino acids long. You look up the genetic code, and synthesize a short stretch of RNA corresponding to that quintuplet of amino acids. Obviously, given the triplet code, this will be fifteen nucleotides long. You arrange the synthesis so that the RNA that is made is highly radioactive. Furthermore, you make sure that, where ambiguities exist for the third nucleotide in the codon, each option is synthesized (see Chapter 2). You now have a radioactive *probe* for the right gene, a labelled RNA molecule capable of binding tightly to the DNA of the gene under appropriate circumstances.

Let us now move to a DNA library which, somewhere within it, has the genetic information you want. Colonies of bacteria containing recombinants are transferred on to a special kind of filter paper, still in their original geographic pattern. The filter is chemically treated to kill the bacteria, break them open, and to separate the two strands of all DNA within them. Further treatment removes most of the protein and other materials, but the now single-stranded DNA remains tightly attached to the filter. The radioactive probe is added. Given time, it 'finds' the complementary, well-fitting strand of DNA and binds tightly to it. Obviously the longer the probe, the tighter the fit, and there are ways of getting radioactive ('hot') probes much longer than fifteen in some instances. After the filters are extensively washed to remove unbound amounts of the hot probe, the filter is placed on to an X-ray film in a dark room. The radioactivity of bound hot probe makes a photographic image which shows up as a black spot on the developed film. The investigator then goes back to the original plate of colonies and picks off the one corresponding to the geographical location of the black spot. It should be the one with the right gene in it. Frequently it is necessary to make colonies sit very close to one another to get enough on to a plate, and one might have to regrow the believed right one to make sure it really gave the 'hot spot'. This method is summarized in Figure 7.

The second method is to get the recombinant DNA actually to work for you and synthesize the protein you want. This involves turning on the switch which allows recombinant DNA to be transcribed into RNA and translated into protein as outlined in Chapter 2. All the thousands of genes in the library are activated; each makes large amounts of 'its' protein. Again, replicas are made but this time treated not to release single-stranded DNA, but protein. Then, an *antibody* to the protein of interest is flooded over the preparation. Antibodies are interesting molecules that the body's natural defence system synthesizes, and they have the capacity to unite specifically with particular proteins. It is fairly simple to make antibodies to insulin, growth hormone, haemoglobin or whatever other precious protein you want. The antibodies identify the colony with the right gene, and the antibodies in turn can be spotted by using a radioactive marker (think of it as a hot anti-antibody) capable of recognizing antibody. The end result again is a dark spot on an X-ray film overlying the area with the 'right' gene.

When screening finds the bacterial clone carrying the right cDNA, the search for the real gene in a total genomic library has taken a giant stride forward. It is easy to make a long stretch of radioactive DNA as a copy of the cDNA, there now being no ambiguities, and this new hot probe can be used as a highly selective screening reagent. Screening the DNA from a million bacterial colonies is tedious, but the technology is improving all the time and the prize well worth the trouble. Furthermore, once a stretch of gene has been identified as being of interest, it is now a relatively simple matter to determine the correct sequence of the chain of bases. If you know the amino acid sequence of the protein, you will soon work out which part of the gene is a coding stretch and which an untranslated stretch or intervening sequence. There are also electron microscopic techniques which can help to sort out introns and exons.

Switching on Genes: How to get Proteins made through Genetic Engineering

It is one thing to get a gene into bacteria, but another to get those bacteria to act as factories for the manufacture of the gene prod-

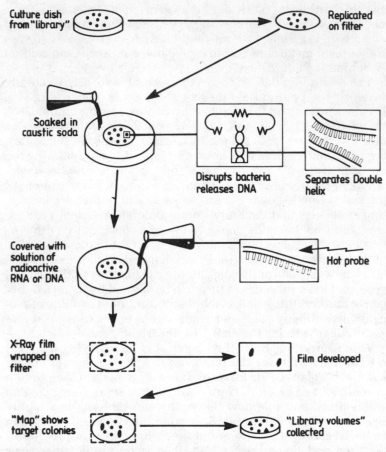

Figure 7   The fourth step in genetic engineering
An example of finding the gene you want: a library of bacteria containing recombinant plasmids has, somewhere within it, a gene of interest. Replicas of all the culture dishes constituting the library are made on nitrocellulose filters. After colonies of bacteria have grown up, the filters are treated with caustic soda which breaks the bacteria, releasing the DNA, which in turn sticks to the filter. The alkali also separates the two strands of the double helix. After suitable washing, the filters are covered with a solution of radioactive RNA or single-stranded DNA possessing a sequence of at least 14 bases complementary to the gene in question. This 'hot probe' hybridizes to specific spots, corresponding to colonies with the right gene in them. The radioactivity can be detected by placing the filters against an X-ray film in the dark. After several hours or days, the X-ray is developed and a black spot marks the site of the 'right' bacterial colony. The investigator then goes back to the original geographical master pattern and picks off the bacterial colony corresponding to the site of the black spot. This should contain bacteria with plasmids that have taken up the relevant gene.

uct, namely the protein for which the gene codes. This is achieved by placing the foreign gene right next to an appropriate control element. For example, bacteria have a complex control system, which years of painstaking research uncovered, that allows them to feed off a sugar called lactose (sugar of milk). As soon as lactose is added to a culture, the gene for the enzyme that breaks it down to the component sugars, galactose and glucose, is switched on. Large amounts of this so-called galactosidase enzyme are made by the cell. The area of DNA capable of sensing the presence of the sugar and of turning on galactosidase production is known as the *lac operon*. It is possible to engineer the bacterial lac operon into plasmids, and to insert foreign DNA immediately beside it. When bacteria with such plasmids in them are fed lactose, they make not only the galactosidase enzyme, but also the protein for which the foreign DNA codes. There are a good number of other operons that can be similarly exploited, and much more refined examples than discussed above now exist. Sometimes the 'on' switch can be thrown by a simple temperature change. Vectors that are suitable for switching on genes at will, permitting large-scale synthesis of protein via recombinant DNA technology, are known as *expression vectors*. Some of these are now so sophisticated that bacteria can be forced to make 5 to 10 per cent of their own weight of a specialized protein!

The Key Tricks of the Genetic Engineer

The key tricks of the engineer can now be summarized. Use restriction endonucleases to break up long strands of DNA into more manageable bits of one thousand to forty thousand base pairs. Get hold of a plasmid or phage vector capable of entering host bacteria, and open it up by restriction endonuclease treatment. Mix the two and use enzymes to reseal the DNA, creating vectors with foreign, recombinant DNA in them. Allow the vectors to infect a large population of bacteria, and use tricks to reveal which bacteria have successfully become hosts to recombinant DNA. Grow the bacteria up as colonies, or phage populations as visible holes, which can be screened to reveal which one has the DNA sequence of interest to the investigator. Then place this stretch of DNA inside a control system that can be switched on and off at will to create a cheap factory for precious proteins.

So far, we have dealt only with bacteria as hosts for recombinant DNA, but lots of other cells can be similarly engineered.

We shall encounter some of these as second- and third-generation variants of the technique.

For readers more interested in what the genetic engineer can do than in how he or she does it, the important thing to remember is that now genes can be removed from their own home in the nucleus of a cell and transplanted in a myriad ways, either just so that they can be studied in greater detail, or so that they can be activated, or even so that their interaction with other genes can be analysed. This permits a near-infinite variety of experiments and of practical procedures.

4

Factories for Precious Proteins

The lot of the nineteenth-century physician could not have been an easy one. A great deal of knowledge about the natural history of disease had accumulated. Diagnoses, though not resting on today's vast infrastructure of specialized tests, were frequently accurately established through listening to the symptoms and spotting a few clinical manifestations. So, doctors knew the havoc that disease could wreak in people's lives, but could do little about it! True, there were powerful preparations like digitalis, opiates and belladonna, helpful in a limited way, but all too often nature just had to be allowed to take its course.

The revolution in the capacity of scientific medicine to intervene and secure the prevention or cure of disease rests essentially on four developments: vaccines, replacements, operations and drugs. Vaccines, which harness nature's own defence system to prevent specific infections, have combined with more sanitary ways of living and have helped to rid the developed countries of many plagues. Replacement therapy, be it by way of vitamins, blood transfusions or hormones like insulin, has allowed the control of diseases where some bodily organ underperforms or has been destroyed. Surgery, including modern obstetrics, can be proud of its many triumphs. In thinking of biotechnology we should look closely at drugs; for it is the large armamentarium of these powerful pharmaceuticals which provides today's physicians with the chief weapons of daily medical practice.

Taken in the broadest sense, drugs are small organic molecules that have the capacity either to mimic or to interfere with some important biological process. Some are natural products, like many of the antibiotics. Increasingly, however, drugs represent synthetic products tailor-made to have a particular detailed shape. Organic chemists think up and make molecules with particular characteristics, say to block bodily chemicals that cause acid production in the stomach, or to mimic the natural molecules that encourage muscles in the bronchial passages to relax. If the idea works, you have a new drug for peptic ulcers or for asthma, though years of trial and error involving lengthy testing in experimental animals must precede any human application. Much of the chemical signalling system of the body, between nerve and nerve, nerve and muscle or cell and cell, itself depends on localized release of small organic molecules, so it stands to reason that other small molecules can be introduced to affect the various control loops, and to put them right where they have gone wrong. The twin sciences of pharmacology (the study of drug action) and therapeutics (the use of drugs in treatment of disease) therefore rest on a firm scientific foundation.

Small molecules alone are not enough, however. There is a further area of scientific medicine which is newer, still uncertain, rapidly developing and full of exciting potential. It involves the use of larger molecules in therapy. Many of these are proteins, and the term 'biologicals' has come to connote therapeutically useful substances of this sort. The need for biologicals can be explained simply enough. Powerful though interventions based on small molecules may be, much of the body's day-to-day business is transacted via macromolecules. Frequently things go wrong that can only be remedied by large molecules, with their greater degree of specialization of function. In fact, some biologicals are not particularly new. We have already briefly mentioned insulin, a life-saving discovery made sixty years ago. Then there are various blood products such as albumin, useful to replace lost body fluids, and gamma globulin, which can prevent some infections, though only for a time. These substances are relatively easy to prepare, because they are abundant, in the pancreas and in blood respectively. The problem with many therapeutically useful biologicals is that they are present in blood or tissues in low concentrations, so that extracting enough becomes a difficult and costly exercise. And, of course, this is where genetic engineering comes to the rescue.

Once a gene for a protein has been inserted into bacteria using a suitable expression vector, it matters not one whit whether the protein for which that gene codes is an abundant one, or one of exceeding preciousness because it is so rare in tissue or body fluids. Properly engineered, the gene for the rare protein can be made to work just as hard and just as fast as that for a common protein. This does not just mean a considerable cost saving in preparation of proteins compared with extraction from natural sources. In many cases, it means an all or none difference—something that was not available at all before is now potentially available in large amounts. Even for proteins that were available before, genetic engineering is frequently a much more practical and sensible way to proceed. Several examples will illustrate the point.

Somatostatin Cloned: the Start of a Long Adventure

There is a hormone called somatostatin, which perhaps enjoys more fame than it deserves. Somatostatin is a small protein, only fourteen amino acids long. It is made in the pancreas and elsewhere by specialized cells, and it represents one of those control or feedback loops of which nature is so fond. Its chief role is to counterbalance the growth-promoting effects of pituitary growth hormone and it also counterbalances insulin, the chief promoter of storage of foodstuffs in the body. Somatostatin will be remembered as the first protein made by E. coli through genetic engineering. It is stunning to recall that this feat was only achieved as recently as 1977. How extraordinary that such mind-stretching feats can appear so commonplace so soon! In those early days of genetic engineering, it seemed easiest not to find the gene for somatostatin, e.g. in a cDNA library, but rather to synthesize it! As there were only fourteen amino acids in the protein, a stretch of forty-two bases would code for the whole lot. The organic chemistry needed to place forty-two nucleotides into the right sequence is far from simple, but it was achieved by the scientists Keiichi Itakura, Francisco Bolivar and Herbert Boyer. They were able to place this synthetic gene into a plasmid vector and obtain synthesis of quite respectable amounts of somatostatin. In the process it became apparent that a few special tricks would have to be learnt to make the technique work perfectly. It was necessary to devise clever ways of splitting the desired protein from the galactosidase enzyme that had been used as the switching device inside the bacterium (see Chapter 3). Also, a fair proportion of the transformed bacteria degraded the newly formed, genetically engineered protein almost as fast as they made it, and there seemed to be relatively little rhyme or reason determining when this happened. Indeed, this tendency for intracellular breakdown remains a major nuisance in genetic engineering research to this day, but it is being combated with progressively greater success and predictability. It looks as though partially completed fragments of precious proteins, made when only a part of the gene has been transplanted, are especially susceptible to enzymic degradation. Also, inhibitors of the enzymes that digest proteins can be added to bacterial growth media. Tremendous strides in what one might term the production technology side of genetic engineering have been made since 1977, and further improvements in the near future are certain.

Human Growth Hormone: a Classical Milestone for Genetic Engineering

David Goeddel and colleagues from the genetic engineering firm Genentech announced in October 1979 their success in the manufacture of human growth hormone. Three factors distinguished this feat from the somatostatin achievement. First, this hormone is fourteen times bigger than somatostatin, being 191 amino acids in length. Secondly, on this occasion the gene was not first synthesized, but rather fished out of a gene library by what has now become one of the classical processes. Messenger RNA was purified from pituitary gland cells, a series of DNA copies was made and put into a library inside E. coli bacteria, the right gene was found within the library and engineered into a suitable expression vector (a plasmid) and large amounts of hormone were made. Thirdly, while the somatostatin work of Ikatura had been *supported* by industry, the growth hormone work was completed *within* industry.

What is the importance of human growth hormone? It is one of the most important triggers for cellular and tissue growth. A tumour of the pituitary cells making growth hormone sometimes causes an over-production of this vital substance. The end result is a giant, with particular overgrowth of hands, feet and chin. Such acromegalic individuals have a characteristic appearance; the former heavyweight champion of the world, Primo Carnera, was a classical example. In contrast, if these hormone-producing cells of the pituitary fail, or are destroyed by disease, the result is what is called a pituitary dwarf. Fortunately, this is a rare condition, and, until recently, nothing could be done about it. Then, a process was developed in which human pituitaries were collected from post-mortem rooms, and, by a laborious chemical technique, human growth hormone was extracted from them. Given the small size of the human pituitary, it is no wonder that the hormone prepared in this way was extremely expensive. Regular injections of growth hormone succeed in restoring the potential dwarf to normal height. In market terms, of course, pituitary dwarfism constitutes a very limited outlet for sales. There is the hope, however, that a cheap and pure source of human growth hormone would allow experimentation with, and eventually use of, growth hormone in other conditions where rapid cellular growth is desirable—wound healing, repair of burns, fractures, etc. This is an area in which one will have to hasten slowly. The central significance of this technical feat is that it showed how well genetic engineering can work in a 'real life' setting.

The growth hormone story also pointed out some difficulties. Early preparations submitted for clinical trial caused unexpected side reactions, including chills and fever. The probable reason for this was contamination by a bacterial product called endotoxin. This is composed partly of lipid (fat) and partly of repeating sugar units and is an important component of bacterial cell walls. Endotoxin is highly toxic when injected into the body—a millionth of a gram can cause a severe reaction—and man is especially susceptible, much more so than rats or mice. At the present stage of evolution of genetic engineering technology, the artificially-manufactured protein is not secreted by the bacteria into the growth medium. It is manufactured and stored inside the bacterium, which has to be broken up in order to release its contents. In the process, endotoxin molecules are also released from the broken bacteria. Techniques of protein purification are excellent, but not yet perfect, and tiny degrees of contamination of a desired protein product by an unwanted macromolecule present in an original mixture can be very difficult to detect. The endotoxin has now been removed from Genentech's growth hormone, but this problem will have to be watched for each and every product of the genetic engineer using E. coli as a host cell.

Human Insulin through Recombinant DNA Technology: a Potentially Large Market

Sugar diabetes, or diabetes mellitus, is really two separate diseases. In one form, which is common enough to affect up to 2 per cent of the population, there is a relatively mild failure to cope with the load of sugar that is taken into the body with a carbohydrate-rich meal. This failure is not due to a failure of insulin secretion from the pancreas gland, in fact insulin levels are normal or even raised. The disease has to do with how insulin is used by the body. This form of diabetes usually starts in middle to late life, is frequently accompanied by obesity, does not require insulin injections, and can be managed either by restricting carbohydrates in the diet or by pills, orally active antidiabetic agents, which cause a lowering of blood sugar levels. The second form of diabetes, which occurs perhaps three times less frequently, is much more serious. It often, though by no means always, starts in teenage life. It is due to a destruction of certain cells in the pancreas which are specialized for insulin secretion. Untreated, it is usually rapidly fatal. Since 1923, when Banting and Best discovered that this historic disease is due to a failure of insulin formation, it has been treatable and millions of lives have been saved. However, the price has usually been two insulin injections per day. The commercial source of insulin is from the pancreas of either cattle or pigs. While pharmaceutical companies have become immensely skilled at purifying the insulin present in such glands collected from the abattoirs, the present approach can still lead to difficulties for some patients. Both bovine and porcine insulin, though very similar to human insulin, are just slightly different from it in their composition. The immune defence system of the body is devilishly clever at picking up even minute differences between 'self' and 'not self'. A proportion of diabetic patients make antibody against insulin, because of these small differences between the animal and the human product. This has two deleterious consequences. First, the antibodies may neutralize insulin's action, thus requiring much greater amounts to be injected. Secondly, when insulin and antibody against it meet in the tissues, a nasty inflammatory response is set up, and so the site where the patient injects himself/herself becomes red, swollen and very painful. You can imagine the agony if this happens twice a day, every day! Thirdly and more speculatively, diabetics even if well-treated get a number of serious late complications, and it cannot be excluded that some of these are associated with the injection of foreign protein. So human insulin through recombinant DNA technology could represent a highly significant advance. Also, from the point of view of the pharmaceutical companies, it represents a far more significant sales volume than the other hormones mentioned.

Human insulin through genetic engineering presented scientists with yet another problem. Unlike growth hormone, insulin is really made up of *two* proteins joined together by an organic bridge called a disulphide bond. Each of these subunits of insulin is made in the pancreas by a complicated process in which the cell first makes a molecule over twice as big as the final insulin and then chops bits off it in a highly organized manner that ensures the correct coming together of the two subunits. Obviously an engineered bacterium would not possess the highly specialized enzymic machinery to do this bit of processing. Between 1977 and 1980 several groups found different ways of solving this problem, and the example is of immense importance for the future, as many important proteins are in fact composite molecules—multichain structures, as they are termed technically. This fact is now no longer a barrier to their successful manufacture by genetic engineering. In fact, suitably engineered bacteria can now make so much insulin that they literally bulge with it, as can be observed in the electron microscope. This insulin is being used in long-term clinical trials. It has been shown to be safe and effective, but only years of painstaking work will show whether it truly has the expected advantages over animal sources of insulin. In time, it should be much cheaper, though clearly research costs will first have to be recouped.

Interferon: Wonder Drug or Not?

So far, we have dealt with proteins, the therapeutic potential of which was fairly well established prior to the availability of genetically engineered material. We turn now to a series of molecules, the interferons, which have excited an enormous amount of interest in recent years, and the true therapeutic role of which will *only* be recognized because large amounts of material are now available for the first time through various new technologies. As so often in science, the roots of this discovery go back a long time. In the 1940s it was found that the growth of a virus inside tissues somehow prevented a second virus from being able to grow in the same cells. In the early 1950s an English virologist, Alick Isaacs, started studying this phenomenon while a visitor to Australia's Walter and Eliza Hall Institute. Back in London, he and a Swiss collaborator succeeded in 1957 in showing that this interference phenomenon was due to cells infected by the first virus making an antiviral substance which stopped a second virus growing. Appropriately enough, the protective molecule was called interferon. Small amounts of interferon were actually secreted by virus-infected cells, and can be found in surrounding tissue fluids or blood. Soon ways were found to induce cells infected with defective virus to make interferon, so you could get hold of a little of the precious substance without doing major harm to a cell; defective virus cannot grow and so cannot kill cells.

This discovery of interferon was hailed as a major breakthrough, because virus diseases, unlike bacterial infections, do not respond to antibiotics. In fact, at that time, no drug of any kind was available to treat viruses. Antibiotics were frequently prescribed for patients with viral illnesses, but this was simply to prevent secondary bacterial infections; antibiotics are useless against the viruses themselves. Even now there are only two or three drugs with proven efficacy against viruses, and each of them has some problems with serious side effects. So interferon was a biological with real potential. But two circumstances conspired to make its development into a real therapeutic weapon, as opposed to a research idea, very difficult. First, interferon is *species-specific*. Mouse interferon protects mice, rabbit interferon rabbits, human interferon humans. This means that all the interferon in the world prepared from tissues of experimental animals would not do people any good. Human cells would have to be grown in culture and stimulated to produce human interferon. This is a serious constraint for large-scale manufacture. Secondly, even under the best conditions, cells in culture make only tiny amounts of interferon. Preparation of therapeutically useful amounts involves massive effort and expense. So interferon languished for twenty years, and not only because of Alick Isaacs' untimely death at a relatively young age.

We owe a great debt to a single Finnish investigator, Dr Kaare Cantell, who steadfastly sought to make increasing amounts of human interferon available for clinical trials of various sorts. Dr Cantell runs a large blood bank in Helsinki. Therefore, he has access not only to the red blood cells, but also to fresh white blood cells, present in blood in much smaller numbers. These cells, appropriately stimulated, are good producers of interferon, although they only live for a short while outside the body. Through painstaking work to improve yields and purification strategies, Cantell obtained enough interferon from these white cells for treatment, initially of some scores of people. Even so, his best interferon preparations were only 1 per cent interferon and 99 per cent contaminating proteins from the white cells. Cantell's monumental effort was prompted by one further major discovery about interferon. It was found that interferon could markedly reduce the size of certain cancers in experimental animals. The thought that something which was, after all, a natural bodily product could prove to be a weapon in the fight against cancer was sufficiently startling to make the enthusiasm about interferon as *the* new wonder drug entirely understand-able. The reasons why interferon can kill cancer cells are not clear. Some believe that certain cancers are caused by viruses and, if so, interferon's action could be seen as part of its anti-viral potential. Others note that interferon can increase the potency of white blood cells, for example by stimulating their capacity to kill foreign invaders entering the body (and thus, perhaps, to kill cancer cells). In that case, interferon might be acting as a kind of booster of the natural defence system. In any case, the anti-cancer properties of the agent provided an enor-mous extra stimulus for intensified basic research and clinical investigation.

Before genetic engineering had its impact on the field, two things became clear from work done on interferon made through standard cellular techniques. First, it was found that there were at least three different sorts of interferon, which were called by the first three letters of the Greek alphabet, α or alpha, β or beta and γ or gamma, each sort having slightly different properties. Secondly, it became clear that none of these three was an absolute miracle cure for cancer. In fact, the anti-cancer potential in actual patients whose disease had spread (or *metastasized*) was quite moderate. It was certainly no more dramatic than that of any one of forty effective anti-cancer drugs that are available on the market. This is not inten-ded as an indictment of interferon. After all, nearly forty years after the dawn of the cancer chemotherapy era, we are still learning about the combinations and dosages of the available drugs that allow us to cure some cancers and reduce suffering in so many more cases. In opposition to most of these drugs, interferon was born under intense public scrutiny and perhaps under the handicap of over-enthusiastic expectations. It has not fulfilled the early hopes, but it could yet find a useful place in the treatment of some cancers, in combination with other methods of treatment. In any case, the conventional supplies of interferon have been in such heavy demand for cancer trials of various sorts, and the costs of production have been so high, that there has been relatively little left over for a major research attack to establish its role in viral infections.

Little wonder, then, that interferon proved to be a wonderful magnet for the genetic engineers. Three different teams announced success in 1980 in the manufacture of various inter-ferons through recombinant DNA technology, and there have been literally dozens of similar successes since then. All this work has increased our fund of basic information enormously.

There are in fact not just the three basic types, but over a dozen different forms of interferon. To the extent that they have been tested, they have slightly different properties both in their anti-viral and their immune-stimulating properties. This means, in turn, that there is a massive amount of clinical research to be done on the efficacy of these molecules in various diseases. The material now available is not just 1 per cent pure, but over 99 per cent pure. It is already clear that the beneficial, cancer-shrinking properties are due to true interferon, not some obscure contaminant riding along within the impurities in the conventionally-prepared interferon. Unfortunately, it is also evident that the nasty side effects observed with large doses of conventional interferon are also present when the pure material is used, and are thus not due to impurities. These side effects, which consist of malaise and fever a little like a dose of influenza, and can sometimes include quite serious depression of blood cell formation, certainly impose an upper limit on the dose of interferon that can be used. The clinical research is broadening out from cancer and life-threatening severe infections to cover separate diseases like multiple sclerosis on the one hand, and simple virus infections like the common cold on the other. In experimental situations, it is now quite clear that interferon can stop you catching a cold from a virus-containing drop instilled into the nose. Will this lead to a nasal spray for wide community use as a common cold prophylactic? The answer is tied up with two issues: cost and side effects. Cost will certainly be decreased in time. Side effects are another matter. They are serious with high doses, but unevaluated following the low doses contained in drops or sprays. Only a great deal more painstaking research will determine the eventual role of interferon in upper respiratory tract infections. My guess is that interferon will have a golden future as a weapon against viruses, but a much more limited one in the fight against cancer.

Relaxin: a Hormone never before available in Human Form

As an illustration of a triumph of genetic engineering technology, with practical outcome yet to be evaluated, one can cite the hormone relaxin. This protein has the task of softening up the ligaments of the pelvis prior to the birth of a baby. It makes the ligaments give more, allowing the birth canal to expand as the head of the baby pushes into it during labour. This effect on joints could have all sorts of implications for the management of arthritis. The hormone is made in the ovary. Until recently, all information pertaining to relaxin came from experimental animals. Through studying the structure of relaxin, and the genes responsible for its synthesis, in animals, scientists at the Howard Florey Institute in Melbourne, Australia, were able to find the gene for the human hormone in a gene library, and thus to work out the structure of human relaxin, and to make it, through genetic engineering. So a molecule about which literally nothing was known beforehand becomes available for study, and possible later clinical application.

Molecular Regulators of Growth

Brilliant though the achievements of the past have been, the future bristles with even more exciting possibilities. As we have briefly addressed the problem of cancer, let us look at one set of examples of great relevance to the cancer problem. There exists in the body a series of hormones that regulate the growth of other cells. Think of them as part of a very sophisticated regulatory or homeostatic system that keeps the rate of growth of cells just right for particular circumstances, allowing gradual physical growth during childhood and adolescence, and then an appropriate rate of replacement of worn-out cells in adult life. Many of these hormones controlling growth act only on specific target tissues, for example the progenitors of the blood cells. Some act only in a local geographic context, influencing the growth of cells right next to them. Most of the hormones are, like interferon, present in blood and tissues in vanishingly small amounts. The purification, and hence the detailed study of these hormones has been a devilishly tricky and expensive task. For example, in our own work, we have had to use twenty thousand mice to get enough of some of these factors for a chemical analysis of just part of their structures.

Now recombinant DNA technology is rapidly changing all that. Several of the regulators affecting blood cell growth and development have been 'cloned' in E. coli and then prepared in pure form and in large amounts. So have some of the factors responsible for tissue repair after injury. The whole relationship of these factors to the cancer problem is opening up. Are some cancers due to the production of excessive amounts of these factors? Or to a cell switching on the gene for its own growth factor, thereby constantly stimulating itself to more growth? Can cancers be treated by drugs or antibodies which stop the growth factors from getting to their target at the cell surface? All these and many similar questions are being posed, and imaginative approaches towards them are being devised.

Growth is frequently linked with a cellular process termed differentiation. This simply means the development of some specialized functional capacity, with the end-result being a non-dividing cell superbly designed to perform one detailed task. Dr Donald Metcalf and his team at the Hall Institute are exploring a novel and rather heterodox theory that they hope will apply to some cancers. Differentiation, too, is controlled by hormones. Could an undifferentiated, growing cancer cell be treated with purified differentiation hormone, to force it to behave in a more orderly manner and, in fact, to give progeny that are of some use to the body? In experimental animal systems we can give a positive answer to this question, but only more work will reveal its relevance to man. Genetic engineering will give us the amounts of factor we need.

Haemophilia and the AIDS Problem

As we shall shortly see, genetic engineering has come in for profound criticism from all sorts of quarters. It may, therefore, be helpful to finish this chapter with one topical example where genetic engineering could get us out of a nasty recent dilemma in a way that all observers would surely applaud. Haemophilia is a hereditary disease caused by the lack of a factor involved in blood clotting called Factor VIII. This can be purified from fresh human blood by a series of fractionation steps, and is now generally available to treat haemophilia. As a result, the lives of tens of thousands of people have been improved immeasurably. However, in the United States, a major problem has recently appeared on the horizon. A disease known as the acquired immunodeficiency syndrome, or AIDS, has been identified and has affected over two thousand people, none of whom, so far, have been cured, and many of whom have died. No one knows exactly why some individuals develop AIDS and others not, but a virus called HTLV III is involved. The disease is commonest amongst promiscuous homosexuals and users of drugs of addiction. In the event, the causative agent appears to have contaminated blood donations in the United States, as a disproportionate (though still quite tiny) proportion of haemophiliacs have come down with the disease. So the race is on for Factor VIII through genetic engineering because the molecule made that way is independent of donated blood. This is a formidable task as the molecule is large and made up of multiple polypeptide chains. Nevertheless, success has recently been reported.

Precious proteins through genetic engineering have fuelled the DNA industry until now. In reviewing the choices I have made to illustrate this subject, I am only too conscious of their arbitrary nature. Wherever I travel and whomever I meet in scientific-medical circles, the overwhelming impression I gain is that medical research into biologicals of therapeutic value has entered an entirely new era with the advent of genetic engineering.Things we had not dared to dream of a decade ago now seem conceptually trivial. Just as well the young do not share our inhibitions! They are propelling medicine into an era the limits of which we do not even begin to comprehend.

This chapter has been written as if the boundary between drugs and biologicals were quite sharp, but the genetic engineering revolution will soon disprove this. It is leading to a very precise knowledge of the structure of biologicals, and of the molecules on cells with which they interact. Armed with this new knowledge, organic chemists interested in drug design are making new drugs in shapes that imitate the shape of the most important part of the biological preparation. Such drugs can mimic the desired therapeutic effect. So a new era of pharmacology has also begun.

5
Genes as Diagnostic Probes

Bacteria as factories for precious proteins have received such widespread publicity that many readers will already have known much of what we described in Chapter 4. It is now time to move into less familiar waters, in fact into uncharted depths where the immense power of the new technology will raise perplexing questions never before faced by humanity. This journey will illustrate how basic research, pursued initially for no purpose other than a search for truth, can lead to profoundly practical end-results. Moreover, there is a fair chance that the next four chapters will err on the side of conservatism. They will describe what scientists can do, and think they might one day be able to do, with genetic engineering. Such an analysis can make no allowance for the entirely novel and unexpected results which will certainly turn up on the way, and which could alter the course of research quite drastically. This is what frightens the critics of science, but no formula has yet been devised that can predict which lines of research are 'safe', in the sense that the new knowledge generated will not be sufficiently powerful to change the established order of things, and which will place in mankind's hands the most awesome powers. These are issues which will occupy us in the final third of this book.

The Nature of the Diagnostic Process

All diseases manifest themselves in ways that give a clue to their nature. Influenza means a fever, a headache, a feeling of malaise and odd aches and pains. A heart attack usually begins with a severe pain in the chest. Appendicitis shows itself through stomach pains and tenderness in the right lower quadrant of the abdomen. By tradition, doctors divide these natural manifestations into two components, the history and the physical signs.

The history is simply what the patient (or the relatives) tell you: 'Doctor, I have a severe pain in the belly'. The physical signs are what the doctor finds out about the manifestations of the disease by a simple bedside examination: if the patient's abdominal muscles are very taut, and he/she practically jumps off the bed if prodded in the lower right portion of the abdomen, appendicitis is on the cards. It is amazing how accurately many cases can be diagnosed by taking a careful history and performing a thorough physical examination. It is also deeply distressing to see instances where the diagnosis of a serious illness has been delayed because of inattention to these two critical components of medical practice. However, and to an increasing extent, such a *clinical* diagnosis is nowadays regarded as only provisional, until more specialized scientific tests are performed. This is not only because an increasingly knowledgeable public wants scientific proof. It is also because most of the clinical rules have exceptions. Loads of heart attacks are 'silent', with no pain at all; some people get the 'flu but do not run a temperature, and an appendix can flop into the pelvis giving different symptoms and signs. So, medical science has evolved a panoply of test procedures, biochemical, radiological, pathological, microbiological and so forth, aimed at establishing as objectively as possible the true nature of a disease and also its severity. And we are now moving into the most profound and, in some ways, terrifying phase yet seen—the establishment of the genetic basis of disease.

The genes—those little packages of DNA inherited when one particular sperm meets one particular egg to create a new individual—always represent a mixture of the half coming from the father and the other half coming from the mother. Moreover, because of a peculiar and profoundly important special form of cell division called meiosis, each sperm in a man (or each ovum in a woman) is slightly different from every other one of that same individual. Take the case of sperms being generated in the testis. These come from ancestral or precursor cells bearing a full twenty-three chromosomes from the father and a further twenty-three from the mother, therefore forty-six chromosomes in all. During meiosis, one of these precursor cells *doubles* its amount of DNA but actually gives rise not to two, but to four, progeny cells. The sperm therefore has only twenty-three chromosomes, known as a *haploid* set, as opposed to the forty-six chromosomes, the *diploid* set, of every other cell in that man's body. Another and even more curious thing happens during meiosis. Before the two sets of chromosomes go their separate ways, they split and join up at multiple places, recombining the mother's and father's traits into new patterns. This happens differently in each individual meiosis, so that each resulting cell has a slightly different combination, thereby creating great diversity within the sperm population. When a particular sperm from a given father meets a particular ovum from a given mother, a unique individual results, genetically different in all sorts of ways from his or her brothers and sisters. Previously, we could categorize such genetic differences in a general kind of way. Now, through genetic engineering, we can examine a person's individual genes with great scientific accuracy. This is best illustrated by a few examples.

The Haemoglobinopathies-Genetic Detection at Work

In 1904 James Herrick described a peculiar and very serious form of anaemia in which the red blood cells, normally rounded discs, turned into a sickled shape. In 1949 the great chemist Linus Pauling and his colleagues discovered that the oxygen-carrying protein, haemoglobin, was chemically different from normal in patients with sickle cell anaemia. This was the first clear-cut example of a molecular disease. Later research showed that the haemoglobin differed in only one amino acid from normal haemoglobin; a valine had been inserted instead of a glutamic acid. This change profoundly reduces the solubility of haemoglobin after it has discharged its oxygen. Therefore, the haemoglobin comes out of solution and forms a hard crystal inside the red cell. This causes the red cell to assume the peculiar sickle-like shape, and often the sickled cell, lacking the capacity to bend and twist of a normal fluid red cell, cannot get through the finest blood vessels, which in turn become blocked. One single copying error or mutation in the DNA of the haemoglobin gene, one base incorrectly inserted, did the damage and changed the codon for valine into one for glutamic acid. That little error condemned thousands to death! In fact, sickle cell anaemia is by no means rare, and we must ask why the mutant gene reached such a high frequency in the population. It turns out that one needs a double dose of the sickle haemoglobin gene to get the disease, one inherited from each parent. If a person has one sickle gene and one normal gene, the person is a *carrier* of the trait but is not affected.

In carriers, one half of the haemoglobin in the red cell is normal, and half abnormal. This is not a sufficient change to allow the red cell to sickle or to damage it gravely, but it does change the cell quite a bit. It turns out that the parasites of the worst form of malaria cannot multiply in such changed red cells, so carrier status confers protection from malaria. Obviously, carriers will not be wiped out by the disease and so reproduce and pass the gene on to the next generation. The malaria parasite was so important in some regions, for example parts of Africa, that up to 20 per cent of people are carriers of the sickle cell trait! The horrible price paid is that when two carriers marry, one child in four from the marriage has the double dose, and thus sickle cell anaemia. This genetic burden was passed on to the American blacks when they moved from Africa to America, so they are now left with the disease problem, but with no counterbalancing benefit as malaria does not exist in the United States.

The discovery of mutant haemoglobins, and the diseases they cause, the haemoglobinopathies, was important in illuminating one of the great truths of Darwinian evolution, namely that a mutation can be both beneficial and harmful depending on circumstances. The diseases give a profound and direct insight into the relationship between a simple genetic change and a severe illness. Since then, over a hundred mutant haemoglobins have been discovered. So have diseases where the abnormality of the haemoglobin is somewhat more complex than just a simple amino acid substitution. Genetic engineering has been essential in pinpointing the nature of the haemoglobin abnormality in many of these cases. The techniques for the detailed analysis of amino acid sequence of proteins are laborious and very specialized. If you go straight to the gene, or sometimes to the cDNA made from haemoglobin-synthesizing cells (see Chapter 3), you can frequently get to the exact root of the problem much more quickly. Also, if you know exactly what you are looking for, you can sometimes arrange circumstances so that simple and sensitive tests can diagnose a particular disease. Consider the following example. You have a hot probe (see Chapter 3) for a given gene, say the gene for that chain of haemoglobin that goes wrong in sickle cell anaemia. You choose a restriction endonuclease that cuts the gene in the part where the relevant valine (which is changed to a glutamic acid in the sickle haemoglobin) falls. The gene for normal haemoglobin gets split by the endonuclease, but the gene coding for sickle haemoglobin does not, as one of the bases is now wrong for the endonuclease to act. So, when a DNA digest from a few cells of a person is made using that endonuclease, and is then run out on a typical size-sieving gel, the normal person's DNA will have two bits capable of lighting up with the probe, but the sickle cell patient's, only one (Figure 8). This stunningly simple test requires very little DNA, nor do the cells concerned have to have anything to do with blood—the mutation will be in every cell, whether the gene is expressed in that cell or not. This principle of testing DNA digests with radioactive probes to obtain altered patterns of gene fragments leads to a general methodology.

Let us now examine the practical consequences of such a technology.

Hot Probes and Foetal Diagnosis

Until recently antenatal diagnosis of sickle cell anaemia, thalassaemia and related diseases was carried out by specialized tests on foetal blood. As there are over two hundred million carriers for the inherited disorders of haemoglobin, and about two to three hundred thousand severely affected children born into the world each year; and as there is no definitive cure for any of these diseases, the antenatal diagnosis is by no means an academic matter. In practice, it has not proved possible to dissuade known carriers from marrying other known carriers. Indeed, most physicians and scientists who have worked in this difficult field have little sympathy for the brave new world in which the priest would say: 'Do you, John, a carrier of sickle cell trait, take this woman, Mary, a guaranteed non-carrier, for your lawful wedded wife?' Not only does it appear impossible to change mating patterns through genetic counselling, but also experience has shown that a significant number of carriers misinterpret the information received at counselling, and are left with the belief that they themselves have a serious disease. Based on those screening programmes for sickle cell carriers that have been carried out, it seems preferable to offer couples the possibility of accurate antenatal diagnosis, and the choice of a termination of pregnancy in the one case in four where disease is actually present in the foetus. I am aware that therapeutic abortion is abhorrent to many people, but the public health problem is so great, particularly in some developing countries, that the option of allowing these hundreds of thousands of mortally ill children to be born and to drain the scarce health resources of their nations as they eke out a miserable existence of a few years' duration is even more abhorrent.

The problem with waiting for a foetal blood sample is that it can only be reliably obtained at about eighteen weeks ges-

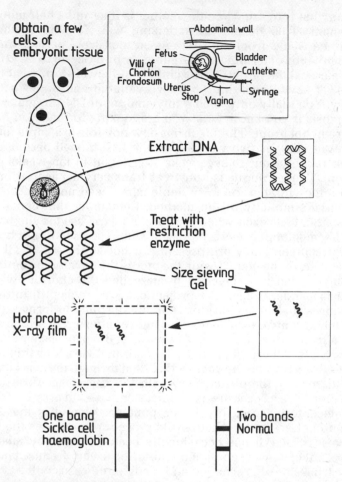

Figure 8   Diagnosis of sickle cell anaemia by restriction endonuclease mapping of the globin gene
In this disease, the gene for one of the globin chains of the haemoglobin molecule has mutated so that a valine is replaced by a glutamic acid. Some cells from a developing embryo are obtained, and the DNA is extracted. It is treated with a restriction endonuclease enzyme capable of recognizing the site where the valine in question falls. The resultant DNA digest is placed on to a size-sieving gel which is then treated with a 'hot probe' for the globin gene. An X-ray is taken, and if the haemoglobin was normal, it would have been split by the endonuclease, and two different fragments of DNA each contain a piece of the globin gene. The hot probe hybridizes to each of these, so two pieces of DNA yield dark bands on the X-ray. If the haemoglobin was sickle cell haemoglobin, the endonuclease does not act, so only one dark band is present on the X-ray, corresponding to the one piece of DNA containing the mutated globin gene.

tation, that is to say when the mother is four and a half months pregnant. This means an agonizing wait for the mother—fourteen weeks from the first missed menstrual period—and a difficult type of termination (frequently by a Caesarian-section-like surgical operation) as the child is quite well-formed at that time. A newer technique is now available and under active study. You really only need a tiny amount of DNA to make the diagnosis if you know what you are looking for and you have the right hot probe. Therefore it is now possible to sample foetal genes as early as two weeks after the first missed period, and quite reliably four to six weeks after (eight to ten weeks gestation). The technique is known as trans-cervical aspiration of chorionic villi, but the formidable name need not obscure the essential simplicity of the method. Remember that genes are present in cells even when they are not expressed in them. So, the haemoglobin genes are present and expressed in red blood cell precursors; they are present but not expressed in all the other cells of the body. Inside the uterus the developing embryo is surrounded by a layer of tissue called the chorion, which thrusts slender, finger-like projections known as villi into the uterine wall. These chorionic villi are destined to form part of the foetal contribution to the placenta (or afterbirth), which also has a maternal component. At the early, delicate stage of pregnancy, a few chorionic villi can be aspirated via a long thin tube that is inserted into the vagina, threaded through the cervix, and positioned by the obstetrician with the use of an ultrasound monitor. The procedure is painless and less distressing than amniocentesis which involves a puncture wound in the skin. We do not yet know whether the procedure increases the risk of miscarriage. It has occasionally been followed by miscarriage; but of course spontaneous abortion is very frequent in the first trimester of pregnancy and many more cases will have to be done before it is possible to say how risky the procedure is for the developing foetus. It is certainly quite safe for the mother. When serious disease is diagnosed as early as this, the mental and emotional trauma of a therapeutic termination by a simple curette is certainly less than that by open operation after the baby has quickened in the womb.

Not every genetic disease can be diagnosed by restriction endonuclease mapping as described above. However, the relevant technology is developing rapidly and aspiration of chorionic villi has already been used for Niemann-Pick disease, Tay-Sachs disease and Down's syndrome as well as the haemoglobinopathies. Many believe it will eventually replace amniocentesis as the first line of genetic antenatal diagnosis.

Gene Probes for Autoimmune Disorders

The 1980 Nobel Prize for Physiology and Medicine was awarded to a trio of scientists who discovered an extremely complex but important group of genes known as the major histocompatibility complex. These genes control a person's tissue type, that is, they determine how strongly or weakly a skin or kidney graft from one person will provoke an immune attack in another person. They also determine immune responsiveness to a wide variety of foreign agents. Until recently, all tissue typing was done by using, as the typing reagent, serum from people who had had a transplant; who had received multiple blood transfusions; or women who had born several children. In all three cases, the immune system would have been provoked into making antibodies against various tissue antigens, namely, those of the transplant donor; those of the donors of the blood samples; or those of the father(s) of the many children. This typing methodology worked surprisingly well, given the great complexity of this series of genes, but it is likely to be replaced eventually by a direct test of the DNA using pure probes for individual genes.

We now have a much more accurate, and rapidly evolving, picture of this genetic region through recombinant DNA technology. It appears that there are no fewer than fifty genes involved altogether, though about ten of these are turning out to be the truly important ones. Simple restriction endonuclease mapping as described for the haemoglobinopathies is already proving itself in helping the further definition of these genes, although it has been in use for less than two years in this area. One of the most exciting aspects of this work relates to the genetic basis of certain important diseases called autoimmune diseases.

The control of nature's defence system is multifactorial, and the immune regulatory genes of the major histocompatibility complex are only one element in a network of interacting control loops. This complex system sometimes runs amok, and the immune defence cells then make antibodies not, as is their duty, against invading microbes, but against some vital constituent of the body itself. These so-called autoimmune diseases include insulin-dependent diabetes, many forms of anaemia, most forms of thyroid disease, chronic diseases of the liver, kidney and nervous system, and different sorts of arthritis, together representing a large proportion of internal medicine. People with certain major histocompatibility genes run an increased risk of particular autoimmune diseases. This concept of 'relative risk' is unfamiliar to most people. It does not mean that the gene is directly causative of the disease, but rather that the person is more susceptible to whatever is the true causative agent. One of the problems has been that the *exact* gene conferring increased risk has not been pinpointed within the broad genetic region of the major histocompatibility complex. Now the genetic engineers have hopped on to the problem. Their first results were announced by Nobel Laureate Jean Dausset at the 5th International Congress of Immunology in August 1983, and I have little doubt that the site and nature of the genes permitting some of the autoimmune diseases will be clear by the time this volume reaches the bookshelves.

Genetic Engineering to diagnose Viruses Gone Underground

We mentioned in Chapter 3 that viruses can jump into and out of the genes of a cell with surprising ease. This is true also for human cells, and when a virus integrates into cellular DNA it usually stops multiplying within that cell, and goes underground, so to speak. Nevertheless, those viral genes can still exert their bad effects on the cell in a variety of ways, for example by causing the cell to make abnormal proteins at the virus's command. Furthermore, the virus that has gone underground can sometimes re-emerge with full pathogenic strength. An interesting group of such viruses is the herpes viruses. Herpes simplex type 1 causes cold-sores, and herpes simplex type 2 the sores of genital herpes. In between attacks, the virus goes underground and lies dormant until reawakened by some event such as a fever, an emotional shock, sunburn, etc. Herpes varicella, the cause of chickenpox, goes to sleep in the nerve ganglia outside the spinal cord, but occasionally comes out decades later in the painful and at times serious condition called shingles or herpes zoster.

Genetic engineering gives us the tool to diagnose the presence of viruses that have integrated themselves into the host cell. By preparing the right kind of probe, it is possible to cross-examine cells biopsied from the human body to determine not only whether a given virus is dormant in the cell, but also, if so, how many copies of the virus have wormed their way into the control centre. This technique can be applied to tissue-cultured cells derived from patients, or, even more elegantly, to very thin slices of tissue obtained from the biopsy and 'stained' with the hot probe in a way that allows a photographic image of the dormant virus to be taken, showing exactly which portions of which cells are affected.

This procedure is important not only for diagnosis of individual patients but also to give us deeper insight into causative mechanisms of disease. Despite its short history, the field has already shown us some important things related to viruses and human cancer. For example, the virus causing glandular fever, an extremely widespread virus which, for the majority of people, causes only a mild and transient disease, is present in dormant fashion inside the cells of two forms of human cancer, namely Burkitt's lymphoma and nasopharyngeal carcinoma. How and why most people get over the virus attack while a tiny minority develops this terrible complication is obviously the subject of very intensive research. Another fascinating example is the hepatitis B virus. This is the agent for a severe form of acute hepatitis, but is also involved in some types of chronic liver disease and in liver cell cancer. In both of the latter cases, some individuals become hepatitis B carriers while a few become carriers only of the viral genes. Again, the diagnostic probe for the presence of the virus is proving a valuable tool for just what is going on inside the diseased liver cells.

The search is on in earnest for viruses in AIDS, the acquired immune deficiency syndrome already mentioned in Chapter 4, and having followed our story so far, the reader will not be surprised to hear that genetic engineering is playing a critical role. One clue, which might eventually lead to a vaccine against AIDS, relates to a leukaemia virus. The leukaemias of many experimental animals, and of domestic species such as cats and chickens, have long been known to be due to a certain family of viruses. There has been a long and frustrating search for similar viruses in human leukaemia. Now, at long last, a genuine human leukaemia-causing virus has been identified, admittedly for a rather rare form of leukaemia. The virus has been dubbed HTLV or human T cell leukaemia virus. This virus is relatively rare in the United States and Europe, but common in some parts of Japan and the Caribbean. Like the glandular fever virus, it can infect many people without doing harm, but in a few, it causes a virulent, unusual form of leukaemia which responds poorly to therapy.

Electron microscopic, virological and immunological studies have shown the presence of an HTLV-like virus in the majority of patients with AIDS. Specifically, a variant known as HTLV

III has been incriminated. If this turns out to be correct, it immediately raises the possibility that killed HTLV III could be a vaccine against AIDS. A survey has found that 88 per cent of AIDS victims have antibodies to HTLV III—showing that they have encountered the virus at some time, though not proving a causal relationship. Less than 1 per cent of healthy humans have anti-HTLV III antibodies. Critics of the HTLV story say: what about the other 12 per cent without antibodies, and also comment on the fact that patients with crippled immune systems become sponges for virtually any opportunistic infection, i.e. the HTLV infection follows AIDS, not the other way round. Furthermore, homosexuals with enlarged lymph glands, but otherwise well, sometimes carry the virus; but it seems that only a proportion get AIDS. So this complex story, which involved genetic engineering early on, is now a multi-faceted problem in microbiology and epidemiology.

Once again, the perceptive reader will gather that, by these few examples, we have really only scratched the surface of genes as diagnostic probes. The obviously genetic diseases are, of course, very much in the minority. Yet a great proportion of human disease has some genetic component. Take heart attacks: one of the most important relative risk factors is a strong family history of heart attacks, but we have only the most primitive knowledge of what genes are involved. The real problem has been to get a handle on human genes—to detect them, to classify them, to study their arrangement and interactions. Genetic engineering has given us that handle, and will alter the landscape of diagnostic procedures so that, in twenty years' time, it will be virtually unrecognizable.

6
Gene Therapy and Cellular Engineering

Genes can be analysed and studied through recombinant DNA technology. They can be removed, purified and transplanted into cultured cells. But can genetic surgery be performed in a real-life setting? Are there prospects for intervening to alter the genetic constitution of an intact, living human being? This question not only poses a formidable technical challenge, but must surely rank as one of the most profoundly thought-provoking social and ethical issues of our times. To place it in context, one must first ask to what extent genes travel around in nature itself.

Mobile Genetic Elements

T. S. Kuhn has become famous because of the theories propounded in his book, *The Structure of Scientific Revolutions*. His thesis, essentially, is that there are two sorts of science, 'normal' science, and 'revolutionary' science. Normal science is what the great majority of scientists are involved in, day by day, month by month, painstakingly exploring all the ramifications of established leads till a large body of specialized knowledge grows up, creating a pattern or overall framework for looking at particular sets of phenomena. Revolutionary science, on the other hand, is that profound shift in perception which follows a major discovery that just refuses to fit into the established paradigm. Revolutionary science, Kuhn believes, is born when normal science is in deep travail, because a generalization no longer fits all the observed facts. The shift from Newtonian physics to Einsteinian relativity and to the quantum theory is often cited as the classical example of revolutionary science, with a shift in paradigm.

I do not believe that Kuhn's analysis accurately describes biological science, which appears to me more like a gradual, progressive drive forwards, with deeper layers of understanding not negating, but expanding, previous insights. Nevertheless, there is a deep truth in the view that exceptions to the accepted rules must be taken very seriously. Fundamentally, the whole of genetics was built up around the view that the genes were the sacrosanct guardians of a cell's or an individual's potential. These genes were inherited from the parents, and that was that. Very occasionally, a copying error occurred, leading to a *mutation*, and this hit-and-miss process was the source of variation on which Darwinian natural selection could act. After genetics was already a mature science, it was found that the genes were composed of DNA. So the DNA was regarded as the stable, heritable material, which was faithfully copied down the generations. In higher organisms, as already discussed, the DNA is packaged into a *nucleus* in the form of separate double-helical strands which, together with certain other regulatory molecules, constitute the *chromosomes*. In these higher organisms, the complex process of *meiosis* can scramble maternal and paternal traits, so adding to the pool of diversity on which natural selection can act.

This, then, was the unshakeable dogma when I was a medical student. However, about thirty years ago, it was challenged from a surprising source. Barbara McClintock, an American plant geneticist working with maize, found a mutation that changed the colour of the cobs. This mutation reversed itself surprisingly frequently, and, without going into all the fascinating technical details, it turned out that what was at work in the mutant strain was a *mobile genetic element*, in other words, a jumping gene. This jumping gene could move about from place to place on a chromosome, or it could jump from one chromosome to another. Once you admit that genes can jump about in this bizarre way, it is not such a large step to the suggestion that they could move from one cell to another. There are about thirty to forty such jumping genes in maize, and for opening up this field, which later was to become so essential to genetic engineering, McClintock won the Nobel Prize for Medicine in 1983. She was the first solo investigator so honoured in twenty-two years. Jumping genes have also been found in the fruit-fly, one of the favourite tools of classical genetics, and in this species it is estimated that as much as 5 to 10 per cent of the DNA is capable of moving around. Chapter 3 showed that genes can move in and out of bacteria, so we have to accept an overall picture that allows at least a certain amount of mobility of genes as part of nature's plan. The challenge, of course, is to understand that natural process more fully and to harness it to useful purposes.

Mobile genetic elements are being investigated in many centres for their intrinsic interest as a genetic system, and for their potential use in genetic engineering as a novel kind of vector. But they are by no means the only approach being actively explored in order to get genes into cells.

Cancer Viruses: How to get **Bad** Information into Animal Cells

So much for bacteria, plants and flies; but can one get new genetic material into the cells of higher animals, including man? The answer is yes, and, extraordinarily enough, the way to do it was first discovered through the study of that dreaded disease, cancer. This section will therefore describe cancer-causing viruses belonging to the group of *retroviruses*, an acronym for the reverse *transcriptase* enzyme that allows them to do their dirty work. The story I want to tell represents the most exciting bit of molecular detective work that I know, and without question the biggest conceptual breakthrough of the last two decades in the cancer field. It is no exaggeration to say that it has cancer research institutes all over the world buzzing with renewed energy as, at long last, we appear to be gaining insights into the causes of this most feared group of diseases.

Cancer is all about the control of cellular growth. It is normal for the cells of the body to divide, but in health the pattern of such division is strictly controlled. Skin cells are shed each day, and are replaced by new cells coming from the deeper layers of the skin, so maintaining the *status quo*. If the skin is stimulated, as by heavy manual work, growth accelerates, the skin thickens and the hands become calloused, but to a degree that is strictly in accord with certain regulatory rules. If the skin is accidentally cut, a different pattern of cellular growth immediately begins to bridge the gap. This new growth stops when the cut is healed. Cancer is an extreme form of breakdown of the regulatory processes limiting growth, so that cellular division goes on with progressively fewer and fewer checks and balances, until the body is destroyed by wildly proliferating malignant cells.

It has been known for many years that certain curious viruses can cause cancers in experimental laboratory animals, though under circumstances that are frequently highly artificial. More recently, it has been possible to use these viruses to create cancer artificially in the test tube. Cells are first permitted to grow normally and peacefully, under good control, in glass dishes. This is the technique called tissue culture, in which the cells are housed in a moist, controlled, warm atmosphere and are fed a growth medium having most of the constituents of the fluid that normally bathes the tissues. Normal cells grow until the bottom of the dish is just covered, and then they stop, just like the cells healing a cut stop when the gap is filled. When a cancer virus is added to the culture, the cells infected by the virus continue to grow and pile up on top of one another in a rather disorganized fashion. They have been transformed into cancer cells. While it is unlikely that many human cancers are caused by such transforming retroviruses, this model system has been widely studied by cancer researchers because of what it can teach us about the basis of the cancer process.

How viruses cause cancer was a mystery until recombinant DNA technology produced a startling new set of biochemical answers. First, it was found that many of these viruses had genes made not of DNA but of RNA. However, the virus forces the cell it infects to make the enzyme reverse transcriptase, which copied the virus RNA sequence faithfully back into DNA. Next it was shown that this copied DNA could integrate firmly into the DNA of the cell itself. The virus had foisted new genes on to the cell! This led to the next major clue, namely that some of these genes were cancer-causing genes, causing the production of proteins which sent the cell wild. Such cancer-provoking genes are called oncogenes, and so far about twenty different ones have been identified, each carried by a different virus. Oncogenes can now be prepared in pure form through genetic engineering technology. These pure bits of DNA can be artificially injected into normal cells and, without any virus involvement, transform the cells into cancer cells. So, in a real sense, oncogenes cause cancer.

How might a gene turn a cell into a maverick exhibiting uncontrolled growth? A few clues are emerging in shadowy outline. As discussed in Chapter 2, genes contain coded information for the synthesis of proteins. It was clearly important, therefore, to find out what sorts of proteins would be made when an oncogene was switched on. A major breakthrough was the work of Dr Ray Erikson, then at the University of Colorado in Denver. He proved that one of the best-studied oncogenes codes for an enzyme known as a protein kinase. In Chapter 2 we met a little bundle of molecular energy termed ATP. This protein kinase catalyses a reaction which snatches phosphate from ATP and places the phosphate group on to the amino acid tyrosine in certain key proteins. This 'phosphorylation' of proteins is now recognized to have profound effects, modifying the cell's growth pattern and its response to a variety of stimuli coming from the outside. In other words, the cell 'infected' with this oncogene has an altered biochemistry and altered responses to regulatory signals. It has since been found that several other oncogenes are protein kinases. Examples have also been uncovered where a single virus carries two cancer genes into a cell. The first gene causes the cell to divide more extensively in tissue culture, but without yet making the cells so angry that they can cause tumours when injected back into animals. The second gene has no effect when injected into a cell by itself, but, in conjunction with the first one, it completes the malignant transformation. This, too, is important, because we know from clinical studies that human cancer is a multi-stage process, with cells becoming more disregulated in progressive steps. The principles are illustrated in Figure 9.

The final discovery, however, is the most amazing of all. The viral oncogenes, or something extremely similar to them, are present in perfectly normal cells! Moreover, they are not only in the cells of the laboratory animals in which the cancer viruses live. Rather, they are widespread throughout the animal kingdom including man! Each of the approximately twenty known oncogenes has been faithfully preserved through hundreds of millions of years of evolution, its structure being only subtly different in the different vertebrates. Clearly, these genes must serve some crucial role in normal growth and development, otherwise evolution would not have conserved them so carefully. However, in the normal cell, the level of activity of the oncogene is very low, and so its protein product is made only in minute amounts or not at all. In the virus-transformed cells, the gene is inserted in an inappropriate place and is switched on very actively. Lots of oncogene products are made, and the cell is thrown out of control. Obviously, aeons ago in evolution, a virus picked up an oncogene from the normal DNA of the cell, and began creating mayhem with it as it carried its now lethal passenger to a wrong destination.

The finding that normal cells possess oncogenes, which are called cellular oncogenes to differentiate them from the slightly different viral oncogenes, immediately raises the question of whether such cellular oncogenes can be activated to abnormally high degrees, and whether this might lie behind cancer as we see it in man. Therefore, genetic engineering has been

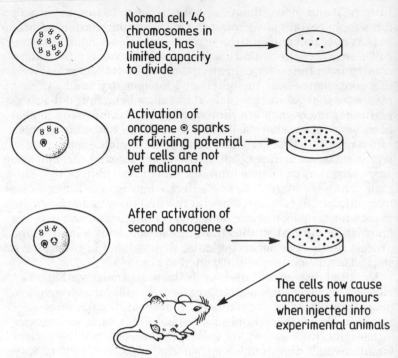

Figure 9   Two possible steps in the development of malignancy involving the activation of two separate oncogenes
The activation of the first oncogene confers immortality on the cell, but does not make it fully cancerous. The activation of the second oncogene completes the malignant transformation.

used to determine to what level oncogenes are activated in various human cancers. Several examples have recently been found where an oncogene has indeed been grossly activated. At The Walter and Eliza Hall Institute of Medical Research, Doctors Suzanne Cory and Jerry Adams have discovered a fascinating example of this. In malignancies of a form of white blood cell called B lymphocytes, they have discovered that the DNA double helix breaks at two specific places. Each of two chromosomes breaks into two. When these breaks are healed, the fragments join up inappropriately. In the process, a particular cellular oncogene called c-myc finds itself not on the chromosome where it should be, but right in the middle of genes, on another chromosome, the proper role of which is to direct antibody formation. There, the c-myc gene is activated to a high degree. While the details are not yet clear, the finding is consistent over dozens of tumours that Cory and Adams have examined, and this translocation and activation of c-myc must be critically involved in the malignant process. Breakage and faulty repair of DNA is clearly only one of the ways in which cellular oncogenes can be inappropriately activated, but potentially it is a very important way for the human cancers, because it is known that most of the chemicals which can cause cancer in man accelerate or promote genetic accidents of this sort.

Cellular oncogenes are present in every normal cell. They do not cause cancer unless they are tossed into the wrong part of the nucleus or are switched on incorrectly. Obviously, nature would not have bothered to preserve such potentially dangerous genes if they did not have an important function in health. It has recently been discovered that the proteins made when some oncogenes are switched on are growth-promoting hormones, rather like those described when Dr Metcalf's work was discussed. Obviously, making too much of such a factor could over-stimulate cells and predispose to cancer. Other oncogenes make antenna-like molecules which sense and respond to growth factors. If a cell possesses too many of these antennae, it will grow too strongly even if the amount of growth-promoting hormone is quite normal. So the story of oncogenes is gradually becoming clear, teaching us much not just about cancer but also about normal growth control.

Tailoring of Retroviruses for Genetic Engineering

Retroviruses have two qualities that make them potentially exciting vectors for genetic engineering in mammals, eventually including man. First, they are usually designed to enter and live in particular types of cells; that is, potentially they could serve as agents bringing foreign genes not to every cell in the body, but only to certain tissues affected by a genetic disease. Secondly, their reverse transcriptase and the associated control machinery could allow a simple linear polymer of RNA to become integrated into the DNA of the cell. Therefore, scientists are currently modifying retroviruses in interesting ways. They are cutting out the dangerous part, the retrovirus oncogene, and putting in instead desired genetic information, in RNA form. Some success has already been achieved in genetic engineering of tissue-cultured human cells by this method. A recent example concerns the serious neurological disease, Lesch-

Nyhan syndrome. This genetic condition, which produces severe mental retardation, is caused by a defect in the gene coding for an enzyme called HGPRT. A mouse leukaemia virus was successfully engineered to insert the normal HGPRT gene into cultured human brain cells. This exciting discovery from the Salk Institute in California will invite many imitations and extensions.

DNA can also be inserted into mammalian cells in other ways. A simple method, called *transfection*, involves just incubating the cells with the relevant DNA in the presence of calcium salts, which render the cell membrane more permeable. This method has a low success rate, but is useful if you have a good method for spotting and selecting the few successfully engineered cells. A technically much more demanding method, which has a higher success rate, involves actually inoculating the foreign DNA into the inside of a cell via an ultra-fine hypodermic needle made of glass. There are also various ways of forcing bacterial vectors (plasmids and cosmids) into the mammalian cell.

In contrast to the late 1970s, when genetic engineering involved only bacteria and viruses, we now have an ever-growing series of techniques for getting foreign genetic information into animal cells. Some of these ways integrate the new gene into the cell's own DNA, though we cannot yet control just where the transferred gene is placed. Other methods leave the transferred gene living and replicating independently in the cytoplasm of the cell. The methods currently available are far from perfect—they should be regarded as evolving. At present they involve a chancy genetic operation, a low to moderate success rate, and quite possibly some as yet unsuspected dangers. But the methods are getting better, and at breathtaking speed.

The Real-Life Challenge in a Clinical Setting

Suppose, then, that it were possible reliably to engineer human cells in tissue culture. What implications might this have for treatment of human genetic diseases? We shall attack this question in two parts. First, we shall look at a concrete example of what might be termed mixed genetic and cellular engineering; secondly, we shall speculate a little on implications further down the track.

In Chapter 5 we discussed sickle cell anaemia and made brief reference to the fact that there were other, related, diseases due to faulty haemoglobin genes. There is a widely held belief that these diseases, the haemoglobinopathies, will be the first diseases actually cured by genetic engineering. In fact, there has already been one controversial attempt to do just this. Martin Cline, of the University of California at Los Angeles, has a solid international reputation as a leading haemotologist, and much experience with tissue culture of blood cells. In 1980 Cline published a remarkable piece of work in the prestigious journal, *Nature*. He took out bone marrow cells from normal mice and treated these cells, in the test tube, with DNA that had been taken from cells genetically resistant to a very toxic drug. The treated marrow cells were transplanted into living mice, and a proportion of them were shown to have accepted the resistance genes—they could grow and thrive in mice given large doses of the toxic drug. Genetically altered cells were functioning in intact animals—Cline had succeeded in a feat of genetic engineering in a model approaching a real-life setting. Spurred on by this success, Cline prepared purified genes for good, normal haemoglobin and treated the bone marrow of two terminally ill patients suffering from thalassaemia, a haemoglobin disease, with this DNA. Further, the haemoglobin DNA was linked to a viral enzyme gene that was supposed to make the altered cells grow faster and finally take over the patient's bone marrow. Cline had been careful to point out to the two patients that the experiment was highly chancy and quite unlikely to cure them first time up. He received their consent to the study. He had also submitted an early protocol to the appropriate ethical review committees. Unfortunately, Cline changed the experimental protocol in a reasonably important way but failed to resubmit the new design to the authorities. The two patients were not cured, and Cline was severely criticized for his (perhaps minor) transgression of the very strict rules governing recombinant DNA research. He lost the United States Government research grants that had been supporting the work, and the episode serves as an example which shows how vital it is to proceed carefully and only after the fullest discussion in a field of such obvious sensitivity.

Since 1980 there has been much progress both in genetic engineering and blood cell culture, and I have little doubt that what Cline sought to do will be achievable in the not too distant future. We now understand, and have available in purified form, the molecular growth-promoting factors that help the precursor cells within the bone marrow to divide and to mature. A modern attempt to cure thalassaemia by genetic-cellular engineering would probably use marrow cells not only treated with the good gene but which had actually taken it up and could be proved to be synthesizing normal haemoglobin. These 'cured' cells would be grown in substantial numbers in the test tube before reinfusion into the body. How could the cured cells be manipulated to outgrow and eventually replace the diseased cells of the patient? There is one way that works, but it is very dangerous. It is to wipe out the patient's own bone marrow cells with high doses of X-irradiation prior to infusing the genetically altered cells. This somewhat heroic procedure, has, in fact, been used successfully for the treatment of leukaemia, where the cancerous bone marrow is killed by X-irradiation, and matched bone marrow from a brother or sister is infused. The main problem with this approach is that such high doses of irradiation temporarily cripple the body's immune system, and in the immediate post-transplantation phase, the patient is terribly vulnerable to any infection. Of course, the leukaemia example is not a particularly apposite one, because, to cure the patient, it is necessary to use a sufficiently large dose of irradiation to kill every last leukaemic cell. In the thalassaemia case, what one wants is to create some empty territory for the genetically engineered cells, so a lower dose of irradiation, killing off just part of the bone marrow, might suffice. As we are talking about a horrible, fatal disease, a good deal of clinical experimentation is justified. However, it will have to move one step at a time, and no good purpose is served by speculating in too much detail.

More Distant Perspectives

Gene replacement therapy may not be dependent on complex manipulations of cells in tissue culture forever. We have already indicated that retroviruses can be modified to be potent vectors for mammalian cells, and it is by no means far-fetched to dream about the day when an appropriately engineered virus is injected straight into the body and made to carry good genes into the diseased target tissue. Admittedly the concept is only a shadowy outline at the moment, but in a decade's time, it could well have taken definitive shape.

There is no shortage of problems to be addressed. Scientists' attention will be directed first at the diseases which are clearly genetic in nature—diseases like the haemoglobinopathies, haemophilia, nervous system conditions such as phenylketonuria and Tay-Sachs disease, and a host of other biochemical disorders. They will also certainly home in hard on the challenges flowing from the discovery of oncogenes. Ways of turning off the oncogene or of neutralizing its product will be sought eagerly as a new approach to cancer therapy. Though it presently strains credulity, one can even dream of vaccinating people against the products of oncogenes and thereby preventing cancer—a dangerous thought as oncogenes clearly have normal functions, but conceivably some of these functions are over and done with in adult life. Scientists will also learn more about the genetic component in diseases like diabetes and multiple sclerosis, though it is presently not easy to see how these could be addressed in a manipulative sense. Other approaches will seek to infuse genes for protein products that are no longer being made by the body because some specialized tissue has been destroyed by disease. Taking diabetes as an example again, it would not be outrageous to conceive of inserting insulin genes and switching them on inside some cell *other* than a pancreatic cell. The problem then would be to design a requisite control system so that the correct amounts of insulin are made at all times, a formidably daunting task. These examples, somewhat akin to science fiction, are mentioned only to indicate that the implications of genetic engineering for medical therapy are indeed very open-ended.

If one were to look fifty to a hundred years ahead, to a period where many genetic diseases were being cured in children and adults, it would be legitimate to voice a concern about the implications of this for the gene pool of the human species. At present, the worst of these diseases do kill before people reach child-bearing age. If the disease were cured through engineering of a particular tissue, say the bone marrow, the person concerned survives to have children, but as the ova and sperms have not been treated, the bad gene is passed on to the next generation. Donning our science-fiction glasses once again, there would be an approach to that dilemma. The fertilized ovum is likely to be a good target for genetic engineering. The patient, then, would have to be persuaded to have children only through *in vitro* fertilization. The genetically cured fertilized ovum would then grow into a normal individual, whose sperms or ova, in turn, would be genetically normal, thus breaking the chain of poor genes handed down to future generations. Presumably a society sophisticated and affluent enough to cure the genetic diseases in the first place would also be in a position to take this further step.

It is important to point out that genetic engineering does *not* seek to address complex multi-gene traits in complex multicellular organisms. The thought that some mad dictator might wish to use the technology to create a superman of great strength or intelligence (or whatever) is out of the question. We know precious little about the genetic basis of the human qualities we value. It is vital not to let our understanding of the highly precise things that can be achieved be clouded by fanciful notions and fears. The use of genetic engineering in creating microbes of greater virulence for purposes of biological warfare is a much more sensible thing to worry about, because given sufficient effort, this might be achievable. As much surer weapons of mass destruction already exist, I am prepared to believe the super-powers when they deny an involvement in such research. Nevertheless, it is important to take mankind's nightmares seriously, and we shall return to these issues in the last three chapters.

A final matter which should be mentioned is that of cost. At the moment, the costs involved in some of the most elaborate things which medical scientists do for patients are staggering. A heart transplant with all the pre- and post-operative care required costs around $100 000. Initially, the costs of whole body irradiation and transplantation of genetically cured bone marrow would not be far behind that. Are these costs so immense that we would be better off making the decision right here and now not to pursue these lines of research? The answer to that question is an unequivocal no. At the beginning, we grope for half-way-house measures that are frighteningly complex, because we do not know enough. As we learn more, we will see that these early attempts represent only imperfect, compromise solutions, and we will find bolder and more elegant approaches which will also be cheaper. For example, if we do succeed in fashioning a virus which homes in on red blood cell precursors, curing their haemoglobin genes, and if we omit the amortization of the research costs, we might have a cure that costs no more than a simple vaccine shot! In the long term, the cost issue should not be a barrier to gene therapy. In the short term, there will be some very tough decisions to make about who will be the patients on whom doctors learn how to turn the bench scientists' dreams into hard clinical realities.

7
Vaccines of the Future

Vaccines are the world's most cost-effective public health tools. Today, we take the childhood immunization programmes very much for granted, scarcely remembering that epidemics and plagues were once the stuff of history: key determinants of the fate of individuals, the winning or losing of wars and the success or otherwise of large-scale migrations. Our memories were jogged somewhat in 1980 when the World Health Organization officially declared the success of its smallpox eradication campaign—this dreaded scourge having been conquered completely by global immunization. For the first time ever, a disease had been totally and permanently eliminated. But in a world accustomed to change, yesterday's dramatic achievements become today's commonplace with frightening speed. So it may come as a surprise that we are on the threshold of a leap forward in the field of vaccines at least as important as the last major quantum jump when poliomyelitis vaccine was introduced in the 1950s. The vaccines of the future will be the products of modern biotechnology.

Principles of Successful Immunization

The immune system is nature's way of defending vertebrate species against infectious diseases. Tragic examples of what happens when the immune system fails are seen in various illnesses, congenital immune deficiency or the Acquired Immune Deficiency Syndrome (AIDS), for example. The end result is death from overwhelming infection. In normal individuals the immune system is provoked to form *antibodies* when foreign organisms enter the body and multiply within it. Sometimes when a virulent microbe infects man, the antibodies are formed too late, and the patient dies. On other occasions the organism concerned has, through evolution, devised clever tricks of evading the host's defences, resulting in a chronic disease like tuberculosis or schistosomiasis, despite the formation of antibodies. Very frequently, however, the antibodies both vanquish the first infection, and leave the patient immune against that particular disease for long periods or even for life.

The key principle which unites all forms of successful immunization is to devise a way in which the formation of specific antibodies (and other cellular processes contributing to immunity) can be provoked without the person or animal concerned having to run the gamut of an actual infection. In the best cases, this leaves an immunity just as good as that enjoyed by a person who has had the disease and has recovered from it. With some other vaccines, the protection is less perfect but still substantial, so the risk of getting the relevant infection is much reduced and the disease itself is less severe in those cases that do come down with it. Vaccines work because the cells (white blood cells called lymphocytes) which make antibodies need not interact with living, virulent micro-organisms. The lymphocytes' capacity to form the protective antibodies is triggered when they encounter specific molecules coming from the foreign invader. These molecules are known as *antigens*. So all immunization involves introducing antigens into the body in a risk-free manner. The antigens soon reach the lymph glands and the spleen and there trigger division among lymphocyte cells, which start to form antibodies within a few days.

Broadly speaking, immunization can be accomplished in one of three ways. The first, which the Gloucestershire general practitioner, Edward Jenner, stumbled across in 1796, was developed much further by Louis Pasteur in the late nineteenth century. The method is to find a harmless relative of a virulent organism somewhere in nature, or intentionally to change a virulent microbe into a harmless strain through prolonged culture outside the body or repeated passage through different host animals. These procedures may throw up a mutant, avirulent organism which can then be allowed to grow and multiply within the body, and thereby provoke antibody formation. Such live, attenuated vaccines work because the harmless relative and the virulent organism share one or more antigens, and therefore the antibodies against the relative can also attack the real organism when it comes along. The second method involves killing the virulent organism, for example with formalin, and injecting it into the body. The antigen molecules from these killed organisms can be effective at surprisingly low doses, as the brilliant success of the Salk poliomyelitis vaccine proved. However, killed vaccines are usually given as two or more injections to ensure that the stimulus to the immune system is sufficiently strong. The third method rests on the fact that one does not have to be immune to every antigen of a microbe in order to be protected. One can therefore inject some *component* of the micro-organism rather than the entire living or killed microbe. The current highly successful diphtheria and tetanus vaccines work on this principle. In those cases, the operative antigen is a modified version of a toxin that the relevant bacteria produce, but in other cases the antigen might, for example, be a molecule sitting on the outer wall of the bacterium. The purer such molecular vaccines are, the less likely they are to have irritating or dangerous side effects.

Principles of Vaccine Manufacture

Until recently all vaccine manufacture has involved the large-scale growth of the responsible organism, or its harmless relative, under controlled laboratory conditions. For bacterial vaccines, like those against whooping cough, tetanus or diphtheria, this is relatively straightforward as bacteria can grow in nutrient broths rather like a rich meat soup. For viral vaccines the technology is more demanding. Viruses are smaller, more primitive forms of life which can grow only inside a living cell. So the vaccine has to be prepared either in living animals (the skin of calves for the smallpox vaccine, or the inner linings of a chick embryo for the yellow fever vaccine) or, more usually, in mammalian cells that are themselves growing under artificial conditions through the technique of tissue culture.

A great deal of technology has to go into conventional vaccine manufacture. Obviously the growth medium must not become contaminated with even one irrelevant micro-organism, so superb aseptic techniques must be used. The workforce must be carefully protected from dangerous bacteria or viruses. For killed vaccines, every last microbe must be killed. For live, attenuated vaccines, the organisms must be kept in a medium which ensures its continued survival, and frequently this requires cold storage. For molecular vaccines, the right antigen must be purified from all the irrelevant material. Quality control procedures must be stringent and each vaccine batch must be tested for safety and efficacy. All this adds to costs.

The Potential of Biotechnology in Vaccine Manufacture

Modern biotechnological advances have unblocked the central bottleneck in vaccine manufacture, namely the need to grow vast quantities of pure virulent organisms. Frequently, as in the case of tuberculosis or leprosy, the virulent organism is very fastidious in its growth requirements. Some disease provokers, for example the malaria parasite, require large quantities of human blood for their growth. This makes mass production impracticable. Two separate biotechnologies can beat these constraints, and indeed are seen by many as competing with each other. The one is to synthesize antigens chemically. The other is to force harmless, easy-to-grow bacteria or yeasts to make antigens through genetic engineering (Figure 10).

The synthetic approach makes antigens in the test tube from simple chemical building blocks. Many antigens are proteins, which, as we saw in Chapter 2, are strings of smaller molecules, the amino acids, hooked together in a particular sequence. The cell does this very quickly and efficiently. The synthetic organic chemist can also, rather more laboriously, build up a protein, step by step, by piecing together the right amino acids. In many cases it is not necessary to inject a whole, intact antigen molecule in order to induce a good immune response. One little corner of a protein, say ten amino acids in length, may suffice to give protection, though, as we shall see, some tricks have to be used to make this work. Whole protein molecules can also be made synthetically from amino acids, but the bigger the protein, the greater the risk of introducing an error into the sequence and the more cumbersome the synthesis. These difficulties mean that, in practice, synthetic proteins are rarely larger than fifty amino acids. Therefore, much emphasis is going into defining 'immuno-dominant' portions of large antigens of medical importance, smaller bits of proteins (called peptides), usually eight to twenty amino acids long.

Genetic engineering, the alternative strategy, harnesses living organisms to mass-produce antigens vicariously, exactly as outlined in Chapter 4. The transplanted gene can be big or small, so that the protein made can be of almost any desired size. Of course, it is still necessary to purify the protein made by genetic engineering from all the other molecules inside the E. coli or whatever other host organism is used. Recently, another dramatic breakthrough in biotechnology has provided an elegant solution to this problem. Antibodies, as well as being protective substances, are also chemical entities of exquisite specificity. Nature has patterned the surface of the antibody molecule to perform recognition tasks in a highly discriminatory manner, so that two molecules which look very similar to

PROTEIN ANTIGEN MOLECULE

THE TWO PATHWAYS

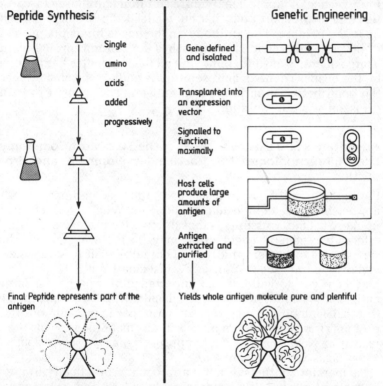

Figure 10   Two separate biotechnologies for vaccine manufacture: peptide synthesis and genetic engineering
Peptide synthesis involves chemical coupling of one amino acid after another to build up an antigen, which frequently is only a small part of a natural protein. Genetic engineering involves transplanting the gene for the antigen into a suitable host cell, as described in Chapters 3 and 4.

each other can still be picked apart by an antibody raised against one of them. The most refined kinds of antibodies are now made in the test tube by taking one single antibody-forming cell from a mouse and artificially fusing it to a cancer cell. The hybrid cell is now immortal and can grow forever, provided adequate nutrients are present. It continues to make the antibody, called a monoclonal antibody to describe its origin from one cell. Once a scientist has obtained a monoclonal antibody to a protein, a giant stride towards cheap purification has been taken. The antibody is bonded to a solid support, for example tiny beads packed into a long thin glass tube, constituting a vertical column. The impure solution containing the protein and a whole host of other molecules from E. *coli* is poured on to the column. The antibody on the beads binds the protein of interest. The scientist then flushes the column through with a large quantity of fluid, removing all the molecules bar the one on the beads. Then, an acid solution is added, and this undoes the bond between antibody and antigen. The wanted protein drips out as a pure solution.

Advantages and Disadvantages of the Two Most Commonly Used Biotechnologies for Vaccine Development and Production

Both the peptide synthesis and the recombinant DNA approaches have their ardent proponents. What is not revealed in many such discussions is that the two technologies are very interactive: genetic engineering may be the way to find the small piece of protein that you eventually wish to synthesize, and testing immune responses against small synthetic antigens may help you to validate the importance of a particular large antigen as a candidate vaccine molecule, which you then make through genetic engineering. In practice, many laboratories probing for new vaccines use both technologies in their research. Nevertheless, each approach has its own special advantages and disadvantages.

As mentioned, the synthetic approach is practically limited to proteins of about fifty amino acids or less, and in fact most work with synthetic peptide antigens has used pieces of eight to twenty amino acids. Intact protein antigens, on the other hand, are usually one hundred to two thousand amino acids long. In nature, these long protein chains assume a highly distinctive and predictable but complex and contorted folding. In the resultant three-dimensional shape, amino acids far separated in the sequential array may in fact lie quite close to each other in space. It was thus predicted that most antigenic sites would be conformational, i.e. requiring the whole protein to display its full shape. In the event, short peptides, particularly those corresponding to the surface of the protein, can be injected and cause the production of antibody reactive with the whole intact molecule. For example, a chemically synthesized peptide, twenty amino acids in length, coming from the immunologically most important section of a particular antigen of the foot and mouth disease virus, was capable of protecting guinea pigs against the whole virulent virus. In fact, on a weight-for-weight basis, this peptide worked much better than the whole protein of 213 amino acids length from which it came. Similarly, short peptides from influenza or hepatitis virus antigens cause excellent antibody formation. While much work remains to be done to see how general this finding will be, recently-devised approaches to *predict* the immunologically most important portions of an antigen through a thorough study of its shape are looking very promising.

It may be, therefore, that the most serious potential disadvantage of synthetic peptide vaccines, namely their failure to reflect the antigens of the whole molecule, will turn out to be illusory. Nevertheless, there is one biological constraint that has not received enough attention. Micro-organisms show a great ability to change and evolve. If a vaccine is directed against just one tiny portion of one antigenic molecule, there is a real risk that the microbe concerned will mutate in such a manner as to change that one component of its make-up, and thereby create a 'vaccine resistant' strain capable of eluding the host immune response, in much the same way that widespread use of antibiotics favours the emergence of antibiotic-resistant strains. To combat this possibility, synthetic vaccines should probably be cocktails of several different peptides, so that multiple separate mutations would be required to achieve immunoresistance.

A second disadvantage of synthetic vaccines relates to their strength as antigens. Living or killed micro-organisms frequently present antigens to the immune system as a bristling array of hundreds or thousands of molecules packed closely together on the surface of the microbe. This, for technical reasons which need not detain us, increases the intensity of the immune response. Furthermore, the micro-particulate nature of micro-organisms makes them palatable to the body's scavenger cells, and scavenger cell-associated antigen is a much more powerful trigger to the immune system than soluble antigen. In experimental situations, these disadvantages are overcome by the use of powerful stimulants of the immune system, called *adjuvants*, which are given with the synthetic vaccine. Most adjuvants are not suitable for human use because of toxicity and side effects. For this reason, interest attaches to a group of synthetic molecular adjuvants that are being developed at the Pasteur Institute in Paris, the muramyl dipeptides and their analogues. However, these are also not free from toxicity. Other approaches under investigation include old-fashioned ones such as adsorbing the synthetic vaccine on to aluminium hydroxide particles ('alum precipitation') to achieve the needed molecular array and also a slow release effect; or newer methods of coupling of the synthetic peptide on to a 'carrier' molecule which is itself a strong antigen. Research aimed at strengthening immune responses deserves to be promoted, as it is common to *all* synthetic vaccines and indeed to the recombinant DNA approach as well.

A third disadvantage of synthetic vaccines may be their cost, which presently is well ahead of that of genetically engineered proteins. It is probable that costs will come down sharply as production technology improves. The major advantages of synthetic vaccines relate to their precision as chemical entities. There should be a minimum of batch variation and of unwanted side effects due to molecules not germane to the desired immune response.

The genetic engineering approach can make proteins of essentially any length, although most of the proteins that have been successfully made so far are less than a thousand amino acids long. Theoretical problems of finding the best *part* of an antigen molecule are thereby largely avoided, although it may still be wise to use a cocktail of different molecules to accommodate the immunoresistance problem. Genetically engineered vaccines need not be confined to one protein—it is possible to insert several genes and have them function in E. *coli*, thus making the bacteria into factories for ready-made cocktails of antigens. The Cetus Corporation has marketed a vaccine against scours, a toxic diarrhoea of swine, based on this principle. The Genentech group have produced a foot-and-mouth-disease vaccine, which works in cattle, through genetically engineering the viral protein VP1.

A further, and somewhat *avant-garde*, advantage of genetic engineering is that potentially the DNA coding for the relevant antigens can be engineered into a living microbe which could actually grow inside the host being immunized, thus making a genetically engineered live, attenuated vaccine with all the attendant advantages of dosage and duration of antigenic stimulation. For example, Dr Bernard Moss at the United States National Institutes of Health has successfully engineered the cowpox virus, the very agent responsible for the global eradication of smallpox, to act as a carrier for several entirely different antigens. Harmless gut micro-organisms can also be engineered to carry non-toxic antigens of intestinal pathogens such as cholera or typhoid, as we shall see. This is an active and exciting area of current research. Because the engineered organisms grow easily, genetically engineered vaccines will probably be inexpensive, except, of course, for the need to amortize research and development costs.

The chief disadvantages of genetically engineered vaccines do not apply to vaccines dependent on living, engineered microbes but to those consisting of pure antigen molecules. First, the need to purify the antigen from all the other products made by the engineered organism, and, secondly, the question of antigenic strength, remain problems requiring attention.

While much of this discussion has focused on E. coli as a factory for pure protein antigens, and on living harmless microbes as gene recipients, there are many variations on these themes. For example, yeasts are frequently used as host cells in genetic engineering, not only because they can be grown so easily, but also because they are evolutionarily closer to vertebrates than E. coli, and thus have the capacity to add sugars to some genetically engineered antigens which are mixtures of amino acids and sugars. Generally, yeasts synthesize and process proteins in a form that more nearly approximates what happens in human cells. For example, the hepatitis B vaccine currently being marketed by Merck and Co. consists of particulate aggregates of a virus surface antigen termed HBsAg, which are present in the blood of chronic carriers of hepatitis B virus, and which have been collected and purified from blood donations. These aggregates are made by the infected liver cells of the carrier. When yeast cells are engineered with the gene for HBsAg, they produce particles very similar to those found in the serum of human carriers, showing that the yeast cell can do more or less what the human liver cell does. These yeast-derived particles have been very strong antigens in chimpanzees, suggesting that they will make an excellent human vaccine.

Animal cells are also being engineered successfully. While they are much more fastidious in their growth requirements, any description of the 'state of the art' technology would be remiss in not pointing them out as possible factories of the future. However, the much greater cost of growing animal cells probably excludes them from practical vaccine manufacture for at least the next decade.

Vaccines in the Pipeline: the Challenges and the Constraints

Given the above technological leaps, it is no wonder that academics all over the world are excited about all kinds of new vaccines or improvements in old ones. Dreams of great daring are being dreamt, extending the concept of vaccination from viruses and bacteria to single-celled or multicellular parasites and even to non-infectious diseases like cancer and multiple sclerosis. A birth control vaccine is the subject of active research. The sky seems to be the limit.

Yet, great though the need and the opportunity undoubtedly are, many academics underestimate the constraints which will ensure that new vaccines for human use will only materialize gradually. The first relates to funding. Vaccine research is expensive and risky, because research and development costs are high; but profits are likely to be low, because directly or indirectly governments are the major users of vaccines, and they are good at negotiating minimal prices. Moreover, drugs are used by patients daily for long periods, whereas once a person has been vaccinated, he or she only requires boosters at rare intervals, so the volume of sales is inherently lower than that of drugs. Human vaccines are less profitable investments for the pharmaceutical industry than drugs, and this is even more the case for those vaccines required in developing countries.

The second constraint relates to the changing perceptions of regulatory agencies. Pasteur's rabies vaccine or even Jenner's smallpox vaccine would have great difficulties in today's regulatory climate, and indeed even the first tentative clinical trials would have trouble receiving approval by relevant ethics committees! Somehow, the balance has tipped too far towards requirements for safety—the risks of not deploying potentially effective agents rarely enter into the equation. Even if this issue is engaged for pure molecular vaccines, and is resolved, the difficulties with respect to suitable adjuvants and any living, genetically engineered organism as a carrier for antigens, will remain substantial.

The third constraint relates to expertise in the development component of research and development. Even though academics are buzzing with bright ideas about new vaccines, their capacity to translate a research breakthrough into a marketable product is notoriously limited, and partnerships with industry will be difficult to forge in this traditionally low-profit arena. Will academics have the patience to see a vaccine through to the development phase, and to conduct the extensive clinical trials that will be needed? This is much less heady work than the original genetic engineering, but just as essential.

It is appropriate now to consider some of the examples of vaccines that appear to be within reach. There is no better place to begin than with a look at possible malaria vaccines.

Malaria Vaccines: Where Are We Now?

There are four major species of the single-celled parasite Plasmodium that cause clinical malaria in man, but the most serious is *Plasmodium falciparum*, which causes the highest mortality, particularly in children. Most of the current vaccine effort is being directed at *P. falciparum*, although if these efforts are crowned with success, the relevant principles will be applicable to other forms as well. Many decision-makers in Western countries do not realize the enormous public health importance of malaria. Informed guesses put the number of cases at two hundred million per year, and in some parts of the world, fifty of every thousand children die below the age of five from malaria. There are over one million deaths annually in Africa south of the Sahara alone. Chronic and/or recurrent malaria poses severe health problems for older age groups as well. Despite notable successes in some countries, there has been a resurgence of malaria over the last twenty years in many others. This is because of the great cost of maintaining effective control programmes indefinitely; development of resistance to insecticides among the mosquito vectors, and the emergence of drug-resistant strains of the parasite. So the traditional methods of mosquito control and drug prophylaxis are losing their efficacy. While it is hard to estimate the economic burden of malaria as such, it is known that not less than US$2650 million was spent between 1955 and 1977 on attempts at malaria control, and in some countries, malaria control efforts consume one half of the nation's total health budget.

A vaccine would be a wonderful and possibly decisive new tool in efforts at global malaria control. There are two basic and not mutually exclusive approaches that have made considerable progress over recent years. The first is to seek to vaccinate against that form of the parasite that first enters from the mosquito's salivary gland after a sting from an infected mosquito. This stage of the life cycle is referred to as the sporozoite. The work of Doctors Ruth and Victor Nussenzweig at New York University has given great hope that a suitable sporozoite vaccine will soon emerge. The sporozoite is covered by a highly antigenic surface protein called the circumsporozoite protein or CS protein. Experimental animal studies of various analogues of human malaria have shown that monoclonal antibodies against the CS protein can protect against sporozoite challenge. The CS protein of the laboratory model has a distinctive and unusual structure, which includes twelve tandem repeats of a particular sequence of twelve amino acids. The repeat structure is the antigenically significant part of the molecule. Recently genetic engineering technology has also found the relevant structure of *human* (rather than monkey or mouse) malaria CS and so one can envisage the sporozoite vaccine being developed either through the synthetic or the recombinant DNA approach in the very near future.

Within minutes after the mosquito bite, the sporozoites enter the liver, and, six to twelve days later, liver cells release the blood stage called a *merozoite*. The successive waves of invasion and destruction of red blood cells by merozoites cause the classical fevers, chills and severe malaise of the disease. If even one sporozoite survives to elude the immune attack, the liver cycle and the blood cycle begin. So malaria will follow. As the CS antigen is clearly quite different from the merozoite antigens, protection against sporozoites does not impede merozoites.

For this reason an Australian malaria team, consisting of The Walter and Eliza Hall Institute of Medical Research, The Queensland Institute of Medical Research, The Commonwealth Serum Laboratories and Biotechnology Australia Pty Ltd, has chosen to concentrate its efforts on a *merozoite* vaccine, the second major approach. While hoping for a 'perfect' vaccine, we reasoned that even a merozoite vaccine that is less then 100 per cent effective may produce great benefits. First, a drastic decrease in childhood mortality should result from a vaccine that decreases the severity and frequency of attacks. Secondly, a vaccine that is non-sterilizing but decreases the average level and duration of parasite presence in the bloodstream would lower the malaria transmission rate in a community, and thus the severity of the public health problem. Therefore, we planned a strategy based on recombinant DNA technology for fashioning a merozoite vaccine.

No antigen analogous to the CS protein is known for merozoites. On the other hand, good evidence exists that anti-merozoite immunity can be protective. It is therefore a case of patiently sorting out which antigens on the merozoite are the right ones to incorporate into a vaccine. We have been able to engineer the merozoite genes for potential antigens into E. coli, and have induced the bacteria to form large amounts of malarial antigens. Moreover, we have devised a strategy which should allow us to find the right antigens for effective protection. Accordingly, we are in the process of testing vaccine molecules in monkeys and work is proceeding in close association with the Papua New Guinea Institute of Medical Research, with the hope of eventually field-testing the vaccine in that country. We are aware, of course, that a number of other research groups around the world are pursuing similar goals. If these efforts, ours or those of our 'friendly competitors', progress to a stage where laboratory studies, including trials to protect monkeys against monkey-adapted human malaria, look sufficiently promising for a human vaccine trial, the World Health Organization will be responsible for the co-ordination and supervision of this work. In the happy event that *both* sporozoite *and* merozoite vaccines turn out to be effective, it would make sense to combine the two into a single, compound vaccine that attacks the problem from two different points.

Hepatitis B Vaccine: the First Anti-Cancer Vaccine in History?

A small proportion of people, for reasons that are far from clear, become chronic carriers of the hepatitis B virus and have large amounts of the Antigen HBsAg in their blood, as already mentioned. As many as 10^{13} particles (10 million million) can be present per millilitre of blood plasma. It is possible to bleed donors in such a manner as to remove large amounts of the fluid (plasma) component of the blood, but to return the white and red blood cells. Further, the HBsAg can then be purified from donated plasma and sterilized. In 1980 a clinical trial proved the capacity of this human-derived HBsAg to act as an effective vaccine, capable of preventing hepatitis B infection. In 1982 two firms, Merck and Co., U.S.A., and the Institut Pasteur, Paris, independently marketed rather similar vaccines. To date there is every reason to believe that this vaccine is effective in its primary purpose, namely to prevent hepatitis B in groups at special risk. This includes people in frequent contact with blood products, such as physicians, nurses, workers in blood banks, laboratory personnel, dentists, etc. It also includes groups such as homosexuals and drug addicts. However, an even greater challenge is looming on the horizon.

Primary cancer of the liver is uncommon in Europe or America but is one of the commonest fatal cancers in Asia and Africa. Excellent evidence exists incriminating the hepatitis B virus as at least one of the causative agents of liver cancer. The *relative risk* of contracting liver cancer between chronic carriers and non-carriers is in fact higher than the relative risk of lung cancer in heavy cigarette smokers versus non-smokers, being 100:1, for example, amongst Chinese in Taiwan. A pathological sequencd can readily be identified from viral destruction of liver tissue, attempts by the liver cell to divide rapidly to make up the damage, and finally frank liver cell cancer. It is evident from epidemiological studies that this progression takes several years. Though the details of how the virus causes cancer are not yet clear, one clue is that the genes of the hepatitis B virus integrate into the malignant liver cell. While the mechanism represents a great research challenge, the practical implications are evident right now. Logic suggests that the prevention of hepatitis B virus infection would prevent the eventual development of liver cancer. One problem is the fact that, in many cases, the hepatitis B carrier status develops in very early life, in the children of chronic carriers, through exposure to maternal blood and/or faeces during the birth process. Thus the vaccine will have to be given very early in life, or else babies will have to be protected by gamma globulin injected at birth and given vaccine some months later. Multicentre trials are currently under way to determine the feasibility of perinatal prevention of hepatitis B infection, and the first results of these trials will be available in 1984 at a major conference to be held in San Francisco, U.S.A. Provided these trials succeed, the omens look good for a hepatitis B vaccine as a cancer prophylactic, though obviously it will be years before a full epidemiological evaluation is available.

Material from blood donors is not ideal as a source of antigen. The current vaccine is expensive (about US$100 for the three doses recommended) and even though two million doses have already been distributed, the thought of vaccinating every child born into the world with human carrier-derived material strains credulity. Therefore, there are at least five or six initiatives under way for a genetically engineered vaccine. The Merck version is already undergoing clinical trials. All these vaccines use the basic principles outlined in Chapter 4, though with various ingenious variations.

Vaccines against Diarrhoeal Diseases

Overall, the diarrhoeal diseases are as important to world health as the parasitic diseases. Perhaps most publicity has been given to cholera, because of its frequently dramatic manifestations and its capacity to cause brisk epidemics, but other causative agents are of even greater public health importance. These include the Salmonella infections, typhoid and paratyphoid; Shigella infection (bacillary dysentery); infestation with amoeba (amoebic dysentery); and a wide variety of intestinal viruses. Diarrhoeal disease can interact with malnutrition and so an infection which might be readily controlled in industrialized countries may prove fatal in the sanitary and nutritional situation pertaining in some developing countries. Oral rehydration and antibiotics are very effective ways of combating many diarrhoeal diseases. However, as it will be many decades until environmental sanitation and personal hygiene practices in some tropical countries reach an adequate standard, the vaccine approach, with its capacity to prevent rather than cure, also has enormous potential in this field.

Yet, the vaccines against the major enteric diseases which are in widespread use, for example those against cholera and typhoid, leave much to be desired. The injectable killed typhoid vaccines are essentially as used eighty years ago. They cause adverse side reactions and the protection conferred is only about 50 to 70 per cent. The injectable cholera vaccine is of low efficacy (50 to 70 per cent) and its effects of short duration (six months or less). Fortunately, research is fast coming up with some alternatives.

On the typhoid front, an oral live attenuated vaccine developed in Switzerland is showing great promise. This vaccine, termed Ty21a, makes use of a stable double mutant of the typhoid bacillus which has lost the capacity to make some of the enzymes required for virulence. The safety and efficacy of this vaccine has been the subject of a three-year field trial in Egypt involving over 32 000 children. No harmful side effects were noted, and even minor adverse reactions were scarcely above those of placebo controls. Over a three-year period, one case of typhoid fever occurred in 16 486 immunized children versus twenty-two in 15 902 placebo controls and thirty-nine in a further group of 25 628 unimmunized children. This 96 per cent efficacy is most impressive, and a further trial is in progress in Santiago, Chile, where typhoid fever is highly endemic with incidence rates up to 140 per 100 000 per year. This trial, which began in May 1982, involves 85 000 children. If Ty21a turns up trumps in the long run, it is a good reminder that conventional genetics can sometimes be as effective as genetic engineering.

In cholera, great efforts to produce a better vaccine by bio-engineering are under way. A live, attenuated cholera strain which goes by the picturesque name of 'Texas Star' is under study in normal human volunteers. It protects against sub-sequent challenge with live virulent cholera organisms. This strain lacks the gene for one part of the cholera toxin and thus does not cause disease. Its only drawback is that it caused mild to moderate transient diarrhoea in 24 per cent of the volunteers, which puts mass population administration in some doubt. Another strand of research seeks to insert cholera genes into harmless gut bacteria by recombinant DNA technology. One variant of this approach towards an oral vaccine is based on introducing the genes for cholera antigens into the Ty21a typhoid strain, and, hey presto!—one has two for the price of one, a combined cholera-typhoid vaccine! This concept is fairly embryonic; it has yet to be tested in monkeys and humans.

Lists, if exhaustive, are also exhausting, and so I will refrain from summarizing exciting work in other areas. Suffice it to say that the above analysis is exemplary only. Vaccine research is alive and well for bacterial infections such as tuberculosis and leprosy, sexually transmitted diseases such as syphilis, gonorrhoea and herpes, virus diseases like dengue fever, influ-enza, viral diarrhoeas and hepatitis A, as well as for a variety of special situations relevant more to developed countries, such as vaccines against gram-negative bacteria which cause infec-tion in surgical wounds. The more the power to manipulate microbes and antigens grows due to the continuing biotech-nology revolution, the faster will these efforts come to fruition.

A Blueprint for Future Action

'Health for all by the year 2000', the stated goal of The World Health Organization, will not be achieved by the six present childhood vaccines alone. They represent a solid beginning for a global immunization programme, but right from the start, the world should be thinking about the power of new vaccines. It has been my privilege to witness at close quarters what two rel-atively modest (in financial terms) initiatives have done for research into parasite vaccines. I refer to the WHO/UNDP/ World Bank Special Programme for Research and Training in Tropical Diseases, and the Rockefeller Foundation Great

Neglected Diseases Program. Because of superb planning; selection of the most worthwhile lines of endeavour and the most able scientists; and a conscious effort to engage the minds and spirits of world leaders of research as active supporters of the initiatives, a catalytic avalanche has started, which is essentially unstoppable. The initial funding has been multiplied many times over as pressure on national and international funding agencies to join the fray has mounted. The conscience of the world is ready to be stirred by this cause. Many of the new vaccines have been waiting in the wings for too long, being largely the dreams of selected, small groups of scientists with limited financial and moral backing. The climate is changing; what is needed is a crystal in the super-saturated solution. We finish the chapter by reiterating its opening words—vaccines are history's most cost-effective public health tool. It is time the world began to behave as if it knew this to be so.

8
Genes as Technological Slaves

The implications of genetic engineering for medical research and practice have received wide attention, not only in the media but also within the scientific community. Great though the medical challenges are, many believe they will eventually be overshadowed by a wide diversity of uses of genetically engineered species in primary, secondary and tertiary industry; genes will become technological slaves. Indeed, it is possible to dream large dreams; anything from vastly improved crop yields to replicating biochips as a revolutionary approach to manufacture of integrated circuits has been the subject of speculation. In this chapter we shall look at some of the issues, bearing in mind that, even with a global enthusiasm for this stunning technology, the pathway from research bench to mass markets is thorny and tortuous, particularly where legitimate environmental and regulatory concerns enter the picture.

Genetic Engineering in Agriculture

Genetic manipulation of crops is as old as civilization, forming the basis of agriculture ever since the practice spread out from the fertile crescent. Any selection of seed varieties from amongst a range of available options is, in fact, a genetic experiment. Until this century astute empiricism guided the choices; but since World War II plant genetics has become a major profession with a regular parade of triumphs. The 'green revolution' which has allowed global food production to keep up with expanding population rests on a disciplined and institutionalized, ever-changing research base. For example, the Consultative Group for International Agricultural Research, a consortium led by international aid agencies, United Nations agencies and private foundations, runs a group of research institutes devoted to improving food production, and its annual budget is $US170 million. Improvement in plants can take many forms: the new species or strain may be more resistant to common pests; it may be faster growing, richer in protein, more economical to grow, less dependent on water, and so forth. One criticism that has been levelled at agricultural genetics is that many new crop varieties have demanded more intensive fertilization, and fertilizers have risen drastically in price over the last decade.

The green revolution now rests on conventional genetics, namely experimental mating and repeated selection for desired characteristics. Genetics is supported by sophisticated plant physiology, a knowledge of the structure and function of plants which guides the principles on which selection will be based. Added to selective mating, astute use of mutations helps plant breeders. These errors in DNA copying occasionally, by chance, throw up a plant better suited to a particular environment. The question is whether genetic engineering can do this job faster and better, allowing previously unimagined hybrid or mutated species to come forward with extraordinarily desirable characteristics.

Jumping Genes: Future Tools for Genetic Engineers?

We saw in Chapter 3 that genetic engineering of bacteria depended on ferrymen called vectors that had the capacity to move bits of DNA in and out of cells. Long before the words genetic engineering had been coined, the American plant geneticist, Barbara McClintock, had discovered that mobile genetic elements, or 'jumping genes', exist in plants, as we saw in Chapter 6. Her work stood respected but relatively neglected until it was shown that transposable genetic elements ('transposons') existed also in the fruit-fly, *Drosophila*. In this insect, genetic engineers have now worked out ways of harnessing the mobility for carrying new genes into flies. One example is a jumping gene some three thousand nucleotide pairs long called the P-element, which has been used successfully as a vector. The hope is that jumping genes are widespread in the plant kingdom and that they will be harnessed as useful ferrymen in economically important plants. In maize, knowledge of the jumping genes and what controls them is growing apace. The trouble is that, overall, knowledge of gene structure and organization in crop plants is far behind the much more detailed knowledge we have of these processes in the simpler bacteria and viruses.

A team that is making rapid progress in plant genetic engineering is that led by Dr W. J. Peacock in Australia's Commonwealth Scientific and Industrial Research Organization. Peacock works predominantly with maize but is stepping up efforts in even more important crops such as wheat and cotton. The research is all aimed, in the long term, at using the jumping genes as a new and rapid way of inserting desirable traits such as resistance to agricultural pests or capacity to withstand drought. In the short term, fascinating discoveries about how and why the genes jump have already been made. Peacock makes no secret of his belief that practical results are still more than five years away, and that a great deal of research and development work lies ahead. Nevertheless, the progressive unravelling of potential vector systems for plants is highly encouraging. Furthermore, a gradual capacity to identify single genes and thus single proteins responsible for plant traits such as disease resistance jets agricultural research into an altogether new era.

Some plants have an extraordinary advantage over animals for the would-be genetic engineer. The so-called dicotyledenous plants can grow from a single cell, so that, in theory, all the scientist has to do is to introduce the desired gene into that one cell, and a genetically altered whole individual could be grown. This is due to technical improvements in plant tissue culture. Unfortunately, most of the economically important plants are of the so-called monocotyledenous variety, and these cannot be started from a single cell. They can be grown from a little plant embryo about 50 cells in size, which could be used as a target for gene manipulation. Tissue culture of plant cells is itself an important new biotechnology. There are also some early hints that it may be possible genetically to transform pollen grains, a procedure conceptually analogous to genetic engineering of sperm cells in animals.

Genetic Engineering and Nitrogen Fixation

Proteins, the nutritionally most important component of food, consist chiefly of carbon, hydrogen, oxygen and nitrogen. The availability of nitrogen in soils is one major factor limiting the productivity of agricultural land. Extensive use is now made of chemical fertilizers containing nitrogen, for example in the form of nitrate or ammonia. As nitrogen is present in such large amounts in the air that we breathe, why is there a bottleneck? To be useful to plants or animals, the nitrogen has to be in a form where cells can readily use it and place it appropriately into proteins. The vital conversion of atmospheric nitrogen gas into potential organic building blocks is called biological nitrogen fixation. Only very lowly organisms, bacteria and blue-green algae, have evolved the extraordinary trick of converting nitrogen gas into the ammonium ion. However, certain green plants have done something equally clever. They have entered into a symbiotic contract with nitrogen-fixing bacteria, in which the bacteria actually supply little factories of ammoniacal fertilizer for the plant. Legumes such as soybeans, clover or alfalfa use this method. Next time you have the chance, examine the roots of one of these plants. You will see small rounded nodules which are, in fact, the homes of the nitrogen-fixing bacteria and the producers of the plant's own supply of fertilizer. In contrast, important cereal grains such as wheat and corn lack these nodules.

The biological production of nitrogenous fertilizers is under the control of a set of genes called Nif genes. Major research thrusts are aimed at the better understanding and control of these Nif genes. The twin purposes are to improve the efficiency of already existing nitrogen fixation, and to devise ways of allowing plants like wheat to fix their own nitrogen. It has already been possible to create strains of *Klebsiella* bacteria that have a mutation which causes them to keep on producing ammonium ions even while abnormally large amounts are accumulating in the environment. The mutant strain has shut off the normal feedback mechanism. Experiments with these organisms have shown that biological nitrogen fixation is extremely energy intensive, and a search is under way for the most efficient species that could harness solar energy for manufacture of fertilizer. One novel research project is seeking to improve an old, traditional three-way symbiosis. Blue-green algae help a tiny water fern, *Azolla*, grow in rice paddies, and as the *Azolla* decays, the fixed nitrogen becomes available to the rice plant. Genetic engineering is seeking to induce the *Azolla*-algae system to export increased levels of fixed nitrogen, thus finally increasing rice yield.

Clever though such ideas are, the longer term dream of genetically engineering cereal grains to give them the direct capacity for biological nitrogen fixation still seems far off. An intelligent policy for agricultural research for the next few years should allow plenty of scope for the fundamental researcher to investigate the structure and organization of plant genes at a basic level. As in all aspects of research and development, the detailed fundamental knowledge will itself suggest new practical approaches. Would that our policy-makers could learn and come to terms with this deep truth!

Commercial Potential of Genetic Engineering of Plants

Though it is early days, the view that plant genetic engineering and new tissue culture techniques will allow a quantum leap in food and fibre productivity appears to be widespread. A consultancy group, L. William Teweles and Co., Milwaukee, U.S.A., recently issued a report which attempted to put a dollar value on the new methods of generating improved crop varieties. They adduced that the present time frame for the selection and testing of a new commercial plant strain, six to twelve years, will drop dramatically. They predict that the sales of seed in the United States, currently $8 million per year, will rise to $6800 million by the year 2000, as by then almost all major cereals, vegetables, grasses and oil seeds in use will be the results of genetic manipulation. It would be easy to dismiss such speculations as misplaced optimism, were it not for the fact that some very large, successful multinational companies are moving into the seed business, which traditionally has been a rather low-key, family dominated industry.

In the meantime, conservationists and other groups have already expressed grave reservations about allowing engineered plants to leave the laboratory or the greenhouse and to reach the farm. This will certainly constrain commercial development, and presumably regulatory mechanisms will have to be worked out which address each category of new crop on a case-by-case basis.

Genetic Engineering and the Production of Naturally-Occurring Microbial Products

It is easy to forget that micro-organisms already produce a large variety of products that are of industrial value. As we have been discussing agriculture, products of use to the food industry come to mind. Vitamins such as Vitamin C, Vitamin D, Vitamin E and nicotinic acid can all be made by biotechnology, and while their consumption by human populations is not likely to rise greatly, they could play a much greater role in stock feeding if they became sufficiently cheap. Amino acids constitute a business approaching two thousand million dollars per year, being widely used as nutritional supplements and flavouring agents. Japan has a high profile in this industry, and an advanced biotechnological research capability in the field. Nevertheless, processes for the large-scale manufacture of nutritionally essential amino acids remain too expensive for routine addition to stock feed. At present, annual world sales of two of these, lysine and methionine, total $500 million. An examination of trends over the last decade clearly shows that these would rise considerably if unit costs came down. Enzymes are also vital to the food industry, being used in literally dozens of processes from cheese production to meat tenderization. These natural products of bacteria—vitamins, amino acids and enzymes—represent just three of many examples where the rate, efficiency and finally cost of production could be progressively and greatly improved by the thoughtful manipulation of the genes of the organisms used. Again, industry experts are predicting that the scene will have changed totally within five to ten years. It could be argued that conventional genetics, too, could have been used for such purposes, but somehow the power and appeal of the new technology has brought a whole series of new forces in its wake. There is a new enthusiasm about industrial microbiology which is worldwide, not confined to the academic community, and bound to impinge on production technology, though to what degree it is hard to foretell.

Further Possibilities in Food and Fibre

Research opportunities in the field of animal breeding and livestock production are currently limited only by the imagination of the investigator, although some of the 'brave new world' ideas may be too shocking for the marketplace for many years yet. For example, genetic engineering of the pituitary growth hormone gene has already produced giant-sized mice that look more like rats, and considerable research towards similar hormonal manipulation of beef cattle is in train. Less frighteningly, much work has been done on improvement of the microorganisms inhabiting the gastrointestinal tracts of livestock, because of the importance of these organisms in the nutritional equation. In some countries, including the United States, livestock are fattened in feed lots rather than on grazing land. In that case, the large amount of faecal matter accumulating in a restricted area poses quite a problem. Biotechnological processes whereby appropriate micro-organisms attack the faeces and digest them, thereby producing usable energy in the form of gas, are showing great promise. Even more exotic ideas are being explored, such as biological methods for defleecing sheep. Here, a hormone, epidermal growth factor, has been shown to be effective, but its costs are totally prohibitive and a genetically engineered version is required to drive these down dramatically. These are just a few of the possibilities engaging the minds of basic researchers. For reasons that are only too obvious, enormous judgement will be needed to see whether a given research achievement should enter the next phase of practical development.

Genetic Engineering in Production Technology aimed at High-Volume Products

The pharmaceuticals and biologicals which are useful in medicine represent specialty products of high value manufactured in relatively small amounts. Amino acids and enzymes are medium volume/medium value products. However, there are also some products required in very large volume, but of low value per unit volume, that have been widely discussed as subjects for advanced gene technology. Perhaps the most interesting of these is alcohol.

Ordinary alcohol, or ethanol, has great potential as a transport fuel. It can be mixed with petrol, 1 part to 10 to form 'gasohol' which can be used in unmodified automobile engines. Relatively small changes to engines would allow much larger proportions of ethanol. Apart from that, the world already uses several billions of litres of industrial ethanol each year, as an industrial solvent and in many other uses. This alcohol is made by fermentation followed by refining. Essentially, three approaches to cost reduction are under intensive research. First, more efficient organisms are required for the fermentation. Imagine the potential of a yeast strain that drove the alcohol content of a fermented fluid from the present maximum of 13 to 14 per cent to, say, 20 per cent or even higher. This would be exciting enough; but what if the yeast could drive the various chemical reactions not at room temperature, or even at blood heat, but say at 60°C? These are the sorts of goals ahead of genetic engineering technology. The second factor in the equation is to find cheaper raw materials to begin the fermentation, including wood wastes, crop residues such as wheat straw, or wastes from processing of sugar cane. Here, also, novel organisms capable of tough and unusual bioconversions would be required. Thirdly, imagination would have to be used to devise cheaper refining methods.

Obviously, there are too many unknowns in this equation for anyone to be confident in making relevant economic predictions. A proposition that is frequently bandied about is that, if oil were to go to $US50 per barrel, ethanol (or methanol) could become economically feasible as an alternative source of transport fuel. Of course, at this oil price, oil shale or coal liquefaction also look attractive, and it seems unlikely that oil prices would go to these levels in the world as we know it at present. But cataclysms in the Middle East could influence the situation, as could major research discoveries in biotechnology.

Many other products in this general category could be listed. Ethylene glycol and ethylene oxide between them constitute a market of some $10 billion per year. Currently these are made chemically, but they could be made by fermentation, and the same applies to propylene. Production of methane gas from wastes could serve as an energy source, and of course in its turn fermentation of wastes could prove to be a major boon for waste disposal. Quite a few biotechnology firms are already active in the waste disposal field. Hydrogen has been spoken of as another energy source which could be derived from industry waste materials through appropriate microbial action.

Attractive though the above examples may be from a research viewpoint, in practical terms most of them seem a long way from the marketplace. Almost certainly, what we shall see is not a blinding rush of new process technology but a gradual seepage of the new thinking into the industrial scene. Some of the glittering prizes eventually to be won certainly justify continued research.

Genetic Engineering and the Mining Industry

It is amazing how perceptions of the mining industry have changed over the last few decades. Twenty years ago mining was seen as the coming boom industry in many exporting countries, a welcome passport to increased affluence. Then came a new emphasis on environmental concerns and a realization that the earth's resources were finite, finding expression in publications such as the Club of Rome's *Limits to Growth*. Further developments of exploration technology and advances in geophysics and geochemistry soon led to the next phase, namely a recognition of vast new mineral deposits, frequently of low grade but of immense size. This, in turn, evoked an interest in cost-effective recovery methods including obvious things like economies of scale but also in greatly improved technology. For most of the earth crust's resources, it now appears that the supply will last a very long time, particularly if extraction continues to become more efficient.

New recovery techniques are relevant not just to recently discovered ore deposits, but also to existing and even abandoned mines. With conventional mining technology, samples of rock released by explosion are analysed to determine metal content. Technological and economic considerations determine what percentage of metal is required to warrant further processing. If a given area of a mine yields a result below the calculated cut-off grade, that particular lot of rock is carted away as waste. The next stage of mining may involve a concentration step, where finely crushed rock is further sorted into the bits with much metal and those with less. The residues rejected from this procedure are called tailings. Both waste and tailings still contain far more metal than a random sample of rock.

With both low-grade deposits and wastes, the question comes up as to whether the metal content can be won in some way that makes economic sense. Here is where some see a bright future for genetically engineered micro-organisms. Microbes can sometimes grow and thrive in the most surprising conditions. The aphorism 'nature abhors a vacuum' is true for biology as well as physics. In biological environments that seem hostile to most forms of life, organisms with strange characteristics can often be found, products of the long Darwinian struggle. So there are micro-organisms that love metal-containing ores, and moreover in their normal metabolism, they often leach the metal from the rock within which it is buried. Biotechnological recovery of uranium or copper through bacterial action is already a reality, and often the metal is actually converted to a soluble form in the process. For example, insoluble metal sulphides are converted into metal sulphates. In principle, these procedures could be applied either to low-grade deposits or to mining wastes.

Some of the bacterial reactions capable of extracting metal require an external energy source. Here, a speculative possibility is that two micro-organisms working together might be the technological slaves, one capable of harnessing solar energy through the process of photosynthesis, the other with the enzymic machinery for bioleaching.

It seems probable that, provided sufficient time and effort were expended on study of the fundamental chemistry and biology involved in these processes, genetic engineers could tailor-make organisms that were better than naturally occurring ones in these bizarre activities. Indeed, recent research on bacteria capable of leaching nickel from lateritic ores looks distinctly encouraging. However, a number of considerations suggest that practical applications are still in the more distant future. Most metals are in oversupply at present, and available at low prices through current technology. Legitimate environmental concerns about release of the micro-organisms on a large scale would need to be addressed and deployment would probably have to be in a phased manner. The mining industry as a whole is much more attuned to physical and chemical technology than to biology. None of these reasons, however, should act as a barrier to continued long-range research.

Slaves to fit any Need?

Some areas of current research have received scant attention in this chapter. A great deal has been done in the area of food processing, for example cheesemaking, brewing, baking and the wine industry. These and the related field of fragrances and flavours are already dependent on biotechnology and clearly capable of further improvement. The chemical industry has grave problems as the major polluter of large rivers. Biodegradation processes could remove toxic wastes from water before its discharge, and could help in other areas of waste disposal. The chemical industry is also constantly on the lookout for more efficient methods to achieve its chemical conversions, where special enzymes could come to be regarded as efficient catalysts. The oil industry is excited about organisms capable of dealing with oil spills and others aiding in oil recovery. Biological control of agricultural pests is an enormous area where true progress has been made. The shopping list is increasing monthly, not through trivial or fanciful additions, but through a permeation of ideas and excitement into the most unlikely areas. Dr Leslie Glick of Genex Corporation has predicted that by the year 2000 the total sales of products made through recombinant DNA technology will be $40 000 million per annum, 60 per cent of this coming from petrochemicals. And A.D. 2000 is not so far away!

Research potential lies at one pole; commercial needs and realities at the other; and in between sits a puzzled and frightened society. The issues engendered by this uncomfortable equation must be tackled in the next three chapters.

9
The DNA Industry

An obligatory partnership links science and technology with industry and commerce. The partnership began with the industrial revolution and reached a new, intensive phase after World War II. It has changed the face of society with breathtaking speed, and in many ways has determined the agenda for mankind for this century and beyond. In 1984, as this is being written, perhaps the most thought-provoking issue in Australian domestic politics is the correct way to adapt to technological change, and to face a future in which microchips rather than people will bear incremental work loads. So Silicon Valley's brainwaves have taken only a decade to become dominant global concerns.

Within the free enterprise system, new technologies are brought to the marketplace through the activities of corporations, frequently helped by government initiatives of various sorts. The pathway from innovative idea to saleable product can take a variety of forms. In the case of the largest companies in innovation-intensive industries, their own research and development divisions may be so large and competent that the whole process goes on within the one corporation. More often, the academic sector in universities and research institutes plays the dominant role in fashioning new concepts, and passes the baton for practical development to industry. On other occasions, individual inventors or small companies drive a discovery a certain distance and then seek the help of larger companies for further development. But in the case of the DNA industry, it appears that a new genre of activity has been born, its patterns a sharp departure from past practice and its *modus operandi* an exciting, if unproved, harbinger of future directions.

The hallmarks of the DNA industry are threefold. Brains are unashamedly the chief assets; research results, in the shape of genetically engineered organisms, are the chief products; and a speculative form of capital raising, termed venture capital, the chief method for financing operations. In this chapter we shall look at the history of this young industry and examine both its virtues and its problems.

The Birth of the DNA Industry

The 1940s saw a great upsurge in research on the structure, function and genetic nature of micro-organisms. Ever since Pasteur realized that fermentation of beer or wine was due to microbial action, it has been clear that microbes are useful chemical factories, but until the 1940s art and craft had been more prominent than science in guiding the relevant process technology. Ernst Chain and Howard Florey's work on Alexander Fleming's discovery, penicillin, changed all that. They showed that penicillin was a wonder drug in the treatment of bacterial infections, but production was hampered by the low yield obtained from the *Penicillium* mould. The first broths in which they grew their *Penicillium* yielded barely one part per million of the precious therapeutic substance. The reasons are not hard to determine. Micro-organisms normally make just as much of a particular substance as is useful to them. They are equipped with sophisticated metabolic control systems which prevent wasteful or excessive secretion of a particular metabolite. These control loops depend on genetic circuitry. In the early 1940s, after Florey took his moulds to the United States, seeking the help of that country's pharmaceutical industry to optimize production, scientists treated *Penicillium* with X-rays. This form of irradiation causes damage to the DNA double helix, and, in the aftermath, faulty repair occasionally supervenes. The slightly altered DNA may manifest itself as a mutant organism. If you X-irradiate a sufficient number of organisms, and have sufficiently powerful selection techniques, sooner or later you will find a mutant that has lost the control loop limiting penicillin production. That higher-yielding organism can then serve as the starting point for further genetic manipulation. This essentially simple strategy improved penicillin yields more than a thousandfold, with corresponding reductions in cost, rendering mass production feasible.

This success ensured that industrial microbiologists watched with great care the ever more intricate techniques being developed by academics for the elucidation of metabolic pathways and the detection of mutant organisms. Japanese industry was outstanding here, making major leaps in the technology of producing essential amino acids. Indeed, industrial scientists were so successful in harnessing mutation-based genetic manipulation that they soon reached the limits of what conventional genetics could do for them. Improved strains could do so much but no more; what was needed for the next quantum leap were entirely new strains with tailor-made characteristics.

The first company that recognized and articulated this need clearly was a small Californian group, the Cetus Corporation, which, I believe, could be termed the founder of the new, élite club that constitutes the DNA industry. Cetus was founded in 1971 in Berkeley, California. Its early aim was to combine biological and engineering capability in a new way. Dr Donald Glaser, a Nobel laureate at the University of California, Berkeley, had invented a machine, irreverently termed 'the Dumbwaiter', which used modern electronic control systems to process up to 100 million microbial cultures simultaneously, permitting automatic surveillance and screenings, thereby greatly speeding up the search for mutant micro-organisms. Dr Ronald Cape (a Ph.D. in biochemistry who had gone on to do a Master of Business Administration course at Harvard University) and Donald Glaser founded Cetus, with Cape as President. The initial plan was to obtain contracts from the pharmaceutical industry to produce micro-organisms capable of increasing the yields of antibiotics. But then, in 1973, came the major revolution. Stanley Cohen's group at Stanford University and Herbert Boyer's group at the University of California, San Francisco, succeeded in constructing biologically functional DNA molecules that combined genetic information from two different sources. Genetic engineering was born. Cetus was ideally placed to enter the fray, as Stanley Cohen and Stanford Nobel laureate Joshua Lederberg, the pioneer of bacterial genetics, were amongst its early consultants. The 1975 Report of Cetus Corporation makes interesting reading. It states:

> We are proposing to create an entire new industry, with the ambitious aim of manufacturing a vast and important spectrum of wholly new nonmicrobial products using industrial micro-organisms ... We propose, therefore, to transfer the genes for human interferon, in one program, and for human antibodies, in another program, into industrial micro-organisms, and to produce large quantities of these compounds in industrial fermentation. To our knowledge, no such programs are under way anywhere in the world ... The opportunity defies adequate description.

Prophetic words indeed in 1975!

The DNA Industry Spreads

Cape and his colleagues were not alone in their perception that a new industry was being born. In 1976 Genentech was founded in San Francisco to exploit the hormone research started by Herbert Boyer, and, from a tiny base, this group has achieved many triumphs. In 1977 it announced the production of the first genetically engineered hormone, somatostatin. Boyer and many of his colleagues were then still university-based, which caused some problems. He later joined Genentech full time, since when genetically engineered human growth hormone, insulin, interferon and many other proteins have been made by this able group.

Another company early into the field was Biogen, associated with Charles Weissman of the University of Zürich and Walter Gilbert of Harvard University. They have done very good work in the interferon field, and have a ready-made marketing outlet for their products. In 1979 the founders sold 16 per cent of the stock to the large pharmaceutical firm, Schering-Plough, for $8 million, creating the first such close association between a DNA company and a multinational drug house.

By 1980 the founding of companies based on recombinant DNA had come to resemble a gold rush in the United States. Though four groups, Cetus, Genentech, Biogen and Genex, occupied most of the headlines in the financial pages, many others had equally impeccable academic connections. Leading Harvard scientists, Mark Ptashne and Tom Maniatis, founded the Genetics Institute. Collaborative Research of Waltham, Massachusetts, was advised by Nobel laureate David Baltimore and Stanford geneticist Ronald Davis, among others. Bethesda Research Laboratories is strategically located close to the huge United States National Institutes of Health and is highly regarded by many scientists there. New England Biolabs was founded by Donald Comb of Harvard University. By 1983 there were 150 small companies in the United States based on genetic engineering and other advanced biotechnologies. Furthermore, most of the leading molecular biologists in the United States now have some link with one of these, ranging from consultancies to major shareholdings and directorships.

Though activity in other countries has been less frenetic, nearly all the major O.E.C.D. nations are making investments in the field. In many countries the involvement of governments has been direct and supportive. Upgrading of the biotechnology industry is major, explicit government policy in the Federal Republic of Germany and in France. Canada, the United King-

dom, Switzerland, the Netherlands and Belgium are all prominent in the field. In the United Kingdom the flagship is Celltech,
which has made imaginative arrangements with the academic
community. Celltech has the National Enterprise Board as its
largest shareholder, but the private sector is also strongly represented, with banks and insurance companies holding shares.
The company has the right of first refusal over any work supported by the British Medical Research Council, which covers
the great majority of fundamental medical research of the
whole nation. Interesting special arrangements between industry and academe are being forged elsewhere as well. For
example, one of the largest companies in the world, the German
multinational firm Hoechst AG, has set up and financed a major
effort at the Massachusetts General Hospital, in return for
which it wins the right to develop the results of the research.

In the meantime, the interests of the developing countries
have not been forgotten. The United Nations Industrial Development Organization, UNIDO, has worked hard to establish an
International Centre for Genetic Engineering and Biotechnology which would aim to speed technology transfer in the
field, promote global co-operation and address problems of
special relevance to developing countries. It now seems probable that the UNIDO centre will be at two sites, one in India,
where there is a significant concentration of first-rate scientists,
and one in a European country. While there is still doubt in
some quarters as to whether developing countries are yet in a
position to contribute to or benefit from the genetic engineering
revolution, I believe in the concept, because such a centre could
help not only developing countries but also small developed
countries, which currently find it difficult to enter this competitive field. As we saw in Chapter 7, recombinant DNA technology will be critical for some Third World health problems.

Australia has made a late and somewhat struggling attempt
to establish a biotechnology industry. Some fifteen or so small
companies are active in the field. Only two of these, Biotechnology Australia and Mabco, which are subsidiaries of larger
firms, currently have a reasonable critical mass and real financial strength. New government initiatives taken in 1983 and 1984
to support biotechnology research, attract venture capital and
provide access to managerial expertise should improve matters.
Australia has a surprisingly distinguished record in basic biological science, and it would be a pity if all the bright ideas had
to be developed overseas. One attractive feature of the DNA

industry is that the capital required for entry is not enormously high. Brains and originality are what count.

Too Much Enthusiasm Too Soon?

There is no doubt that the prospects for the DNA industry have often been the subject of considerable hyperbole. Let us return to the United States pioneers and see how they have financed the developmental research for which they have become famous. The most highly publicized example is Genentech. It now employs about 350 people including seventy Ph.D.s and its annual research expenditure is over $20 million. Where do these funds come from? Back in 1977 Robert Swanson, the President, had raised nearly $1 million for Genentech from sources such as International Nickel Co. and the venture capital firm, Kleiner and Perkins. It seemed an enormous amount at the time! By 1980 the company had grown to the degree that a public offering of stock seemed appropriate. A million shares were offered at $35 each, but the providers of this $35 million ended up with only 13 per cent of the company! Yet, on the first day's trading, the shares shot up (briefly) to $89! At one stage, Wall Street was theoretically valuing the company at over half a billion dollars and Herbert Boyer's original investment of a few hundred dollars had a paper value of $80 million. For comparison, the Upjohn Company, one of the leading, established pharmaceutical firms, had a market capitalization of $1 billion. This excessive enthusiasm did not last long, and Genentech stock settled back to its issue price. When Schering Plough bought 16 per cent of Biogen in 1979 this set a paper value for the group of $50 million and by 1980 Biogen was looking for more capital on the basis of a self-assessed value of $100 million. At the time, the firm was employing a total of sixteen scientists in its laboratory in Geneva, and had not generated any sales revenue!

The Cetus Corporation went public only in 1981, offering its stock for $23 per share. The capital raising of $120 million was a record for a flotation of this type. As a result, Cetus now has five hundred employees and an operating expenditure budget of $30 million a year. Its product sales and research-associated revenues for 1983 were $18½ million, and interest on the capital raised brought it close to break-even point for the year. Cetus's intention is to operate at a small profit in the next few years, and its directors are confident that, as new products in health care, agricultural and veterinary science and industrial applications reach the market, Cetus will fully justify its market value on conventional criteria.

Perhaps the scale of access to venture capital just discussed, and the degree of equity dilution which the later waves of investors appear prepared to accept, are peculiarly American characteristics. Nevertheless, a substantial amount of private capital has also been expended in other countries. It seems likely that many of the smaller DNA companies will fail. The real question is whether those that do succeed will reap rewards for their shareholders commensurate with the risks that have been taken. Certainly the total world market for the products coming forward are potentially enormous, but these new specialty companies face several real problems. First, gene cloning technology is constantly improving and much of the new knowledge will remain in the public domain, making it possible for competitors to catch up quickly. Secondly, patents in this area will be difficult to defend. Thirdly, and perhaps most importantly, many new companies do not have either the experience in production technology and scale-up of larger, older companies or established skills in marketing. It seems inevitable that, in most cases, links of one sort or another will have to be developed with established larger corporations. With considerably less fuss, many of the leading drug firms, such as Eli Lilly or Hoffmann-la Roche, have added skills in genetic engineering to their own in-house research expertise, and their greater experience with the regulatory procedures imposed by governments before products can be sold gives them a major advantage. Yet I believe the best venture capital firms will succeed and represent an important and beneficial adventure.

The Role of the DNA Industry in Academic Biology

The real achievement of firms like Cetus and Genentech has been to forge a new alliance between industry and the academic community. There have, of course, been reasonably close relationships between these worlds in other branches of medical science. Departments of Pharmacology in medical schools interact widely with manufacturers of ethical pharmaceuticals. On the whole, however, a rather subtle and not altogether worthy tension has surrounded this relationship. Frequently, the best medical scientists have ended up in universities and research institutes and have looked down somewhat on those of their colleagues who have gone to industry. Some academics have gone even further and regarded drug companies as little more than milking cows, good for providing money in their research, but otherwise of little worth. In departments of bio-chemistry, genetics, microbiology or immunology, knowledge of industry was minimal and contacts confined to a few particular instances. What the new DNA firms did was to bring a new and much more free-wheeling atmosphere to the industrial research laboratory. Scientists working for these companies say that they do not *feel* confined; the ebb and flow of discussion and the looseness of administrative controls resemble the atmosphere of a university. This has proved attractive to many good young minds.

The stellar character of some of the entrepreneurs also helped. If a Donald Glaser, a Herbert Boyer or a Walter Gilbert backed a venture, could it be anything other than exciting and worth while? The scientific advisory boards played their part—in fact, in some cases, they were even more luminary than the scientific advisory boards of the purest of the élite research institutes! Associates of the better firms started sending some of their *best* post-doctoral fellows into the DNA industry, not, as had been the case in the past, the weaker ones who would not quite 'make it' on the academic scene. So excellence became the norm and, as in the universities themselves, a self-perpetuating element. Scientists began to realize they could be rich *and* famous—this was something new and strange. It is worth adding that over the last decade as university finances have tightened, the established pharmaceutical industry itself is also attracting some excellent research stars.

Shifts in perception as basic as this do not occur without much trauma. Turmoil and unease has swept through the universities as a result of the birth of the DNA industry, and some of the worries are real. The chief ones relate to conflict of interest and secrecy. All over the world, academics draw their main support from government grants; in other words, from taxation dollars. In a real sense, therefore, the creativity of academics, who are relatively well paid and, in many instances, securely employed, should benefit the whole community. Yet when a breakthrough of potential importance to industry occurs, there is the temptation to derive some personal gain or benefit from it. Different institutions approach this problem in different ways. In Australia, for example, it is the norm to regard all patentable discoveries as belonging to the employing institution, which in fact takes out the patent and derives the ultimate financial advantage. This is regarded as fair, because the institution has borne the costs and assumed the risks of the research. The institution itself frequently has to share its rights with a governmental granting agency. Furthermore, the inventor will gain indirectly through prestige, promotion and perhaps greater security of tenure. In most institutions the scientist is allowed to augment his or her income by a small percentage through consulting, and this gives further opportunities to some better-known workers.

In the United States a more entrepreneurial spirit exists, and many universities allow academics to retain a proportion of the patent rights of their discovery for themselves. Usually this proportion is moderate, say 15 to 33 per cent. This is seen as giving individual scientists more incentive to think about the eventual practical implications of their work. The universities take a very stern view of scientists who achieve a development while working as academics under a grant, and then promptly take their discovery, for example a genetically engineered clone, and join a venture capital firm. This has already been the subject of lawsuits in the United States; however, the practice is very hard to police and doubtless there are many marginal cases where part of a discovery was made in a university laboratory and part after the move to industry.

There is great dissension over the question of whether a professor can work simultaneously for a university and directly within a venture capital firm (as distinct from consulting with it). Some universities regard this as perfectly acceptable, provided the university knows of, and has approved, the arrangement. Others forbid the practice and insist that the conflict of interest would then be too great—the scientist is forced to choose between his old loyalties and peer group and the new potential prizes. Again there are no clear-cut rights and wrongs in the situation; so much will depend on the cultural norms of the society concerned, and the personal integrity of the individuals.

A creeping secrecy within molecular biology represents a real threat. This discipline has a glorious tradition of openness, ideas flying across the oceans at great speed, and competition relating more to brilliance of insight and elegance of experimentation than to thoughts of financial reward. This tradition is beautifully described in Horace Judson's *The Eighth Day of Creation*. Yet it is being eroded, and may even be destroyed through the boom in genetic engineering. Scientists who were once so eager for their few minutes in the limelight within the peer group are turning coy at the large international conferences, skirting over details and even refusing point blank to reveal technical or structural data. This is destructive of progress in molecular biology which has depended not just on the sharing of concepts but also on trenchantly strict peer group criticism of techniques and results. A new sequence seen with increasing frequency is: discover, patent, call a press conference to boost your stock, then publish! Irksome though it may seem, this is still much better than the norm in some industries, where publication is delayed for months or even years for commercial reasons. Despite present trends, I am not as pessimistic as some about the death of the normal academic tradition of free exchange of information. The motivation to shine in the eyes of one's most distinguished colleagues is still very strong among scientists, and good lectures at conferences plus first-class written papers are still the best ways of achieving that peer group esteem which is so treasured.

An Orderly Future for the DNA Industry

I predict a more orderly, if pluralistic, development of the DNA industry in the 1980s and 1990s. I have no doubt that the fundamental technology of gene cloning and expression will continue to develop with amazing speed and to dominate biomedical science over this period. However, workers in the DNA industry will not just be recipients of this technology; they will increasingly contribute to it. Many of the smaller DNA companies will disappear and others will merge with more successful members of the club. Some DNA companies will be taken over by pharmaceutical or other multinational firms. In general, large enterprises in drugs and biologicals, the food industry, agriculture, the extractive industries and the chemical industry will greatly expand their own capabilities in molecular and cell biology and genetics, and in time this total research base will exceed the specialty companies in size, though probably not in quality.

Government initiatives will ensure considerable international competitiveness in biotechnology, and a rapid overall growth of the industry. The demarcation between genetic engineering and other biologically-based process technologies will steadily diminish. Genetic engineering will come to be seen as one of many possible options for problem solving. As this happens, the almost mystical aura that now surrounds the field will fade. The 'hype' will diminish, the special government programmes will be subsumed into the normal mechanisms for industry incentives, and market forces will assert themselves, ensuring the success of the best lines of research and the failure of many others.

Eventually, we shall be grateful for the present phase of the DNA industry. Though it will pass into history characterized by many exaggerations, it has been one force responsible for drawing increased attention to the immense power of biological science, now that the gene is understood. In the end, we shall be more glad than sorry that the academic sector had to confront mammon in this special new way. The contract between society and its institutions of higher learning has never been an easy one, and shared practical goals are one important way of bridging the gulf. I look forward to the day when scientists will move easily between academe and industry—and back again—enlarging the contacts, softening the hard edges of misunderstanding and mistrust. Such untidy pluralism will allow the best brains to be challenged and stretched to the greatest extent, for the betterment of mankind.

10
Scientists Playing God

How far should scientists go in exploring the secrets of life? Who should decide what is an ethical and safe experiment? What concerns should influence a decision to move from laboratory bench to commercial application or clinical practice? Above all, how will the awesome power to manipulate the very fabric of life affect mankind's perception of the universe and man's place in it? These are just a few of the ethical, moral and philosophical issues arising from genetic engineering. None of them are entirely new, but the intensity with which they are being raised and the widespread nature of the debate exceed anything witnessed previously for the biological sciences. The picture is reminiscent of the agony of the atomic scientists nearly forty years ago.

There are some similarities, but also some striking differences. Nuclear physics was born in a quiet, protected academic environment and grew up in the secrecy imposed by a world war. Genetic engineering has been the subject of intense societal scrutiny from the time that it was no more than a boffin's pipe-dream. Moreover, it was the scientists themselves who sounded the alarm, and the history of the early worries is worth reviewing.

A Unique Voluntary Moratorium

The biochemists chiefly responsible for forging the molecular biology revolution spring from a different background and possess different skills from the traditional medical microbiologists who isolate disease organisms and learn how to handle these safely. Accordingly, it was not surprising that when animal viruses and mammalian cultured cells became popular tools, the molecular biologists began to worry about laboratory safety. In fact, in January 1973, a meeting was held in Asilomar,

California, to debate the biohazards of certain kinds of virus work, but curiously neither this conference nor the book published from it occasioned media comment or other lay interest. By June of the same year, things had moved faster than anyone had expected. The extraordinary power of the restriction endonucleases (Chapter 3) which permit precise excision of genes came into full focus, and the first recombined DNA molecules became a reality. The relevant results were discussed at a Gordon Conference in the United States, and the participants at this meeting voted to express publicly their concern about potential risks. This was done by way of a letter sent to the Presidents of the United States National Academy of Sciences and National Institute of Medicine which was published in the widely-read magazine, Science, in September 1973.

This initial letter was phrased with great care; its arguments have stood the test of the intervening eleven years. It describes the technical ability to join together DNA molecules from diverse sources, and gives, as an example, the fusion of viral and bacterial DNA. It urges the Academies to establish a committee to study possible hazards, which, however, are firmly flagged as conjectural. Despite major articles in Science and The New Scientist, public reaction was still muted. An Academy Committee was set up to examine potential hazards of genetic engineering. It was under the chairmanship of Dr Paul Berg, one of the pioneers of gene splicing, who was later to receive a Nobel Prize.

This committee published some of its key recommendations in Science in July 1974. This has come to be referred to as the 'Berg letter'. By that time, both phages and plasmids were working as vectors for recombined genes. Some scientists were deeply worried that the commonest host bacterium was E. coli, a resident of the human intestine. What if a recombined organism, carrying, for example, genes from a cancer-causing virus, were to escape from the laboratory and spread like a plague? Could an epidemic of cancer result? Faced with such awesome hypotheses, the Berg committee called for a voluntary world moratorium on certain defined experiments deemed to be hazardous; recommended the establishment of a recombinant DNA monitoring committee within the United States National Institutes of Health; and foreshadowed a representative international meeting in 1975 to review the situation.

The Berg letter is historic, not only because of the gravity of its subject-matter, but also because it represents the first time that a senior, responsible group of biologists has called for the voluntary deferral of experiments, some of which were of extraordinary potential interest. Furthermore, until that time, concerns had been kept largely within 'the club', but now the world at large was invited to share it. Now that the cat was out of the bag, press comment accelerated markedly, particularly in New York and Washington. As far as can be determined, the moratorium was obeyed within the United States.

Most of the early genetic engineering technology had been developed in the United States, but the clever tricks were easy to copy so the reaction of European scientists was watched with great interest. They had no fiscal reason to follow a United States-based moratorium. Whereas a researcher breaking the rules in the United States faced curtailment of grant funding, moral suasion across the Atlantic was the only way Europe could be influenced. Predictably, reaction to the Berg letter in Europe was distinctly mixed. Some leaders obeyed the moratorium; a few others kept working away without making too much noise about it. In the event, the United Kingdom took the lead under the chairmanship of Lord Ashby and set up a high-powered working party, which published some eminently sensible and not unduly restrictive recommendations in January 1975. Nevertheless, it is probable that the moratorium in the United States, which lasted from July 1974 to February 1975, allowed European molecular biologists to catch up at least a little in a field which was moving with dramatic speed.

Asilomar was, once again, chosen as the site of the major international forum at which the whole world could debate genetic engineering. The world of biology really proved its solidarity at Asilomar. Most of the developed countries, including the Soviet Union, sent their top scientists; and both the press and the legal profession were amply represented. After six days of scientific presentations and vigorous discussion, a consensus document was approved with only a very few dissenting votes. The conference decided to lift the moratorium and to provide a stringent set of guidelines so that experiments could be pursued safely. It recommended two types of containment of recombined organisms; biological containment, which means disabling the host bacteria or the recombinant vectors in such a way as to make it impossible for them to survive in anything other than an artificial laboratory environment; and physical containment preventing the exit of microbes from the laboratory where the research was being performed. The types of containment recommended varied among experiments considered of minimal risk, low risk, moderate risk or high risk. Special laboratories designated P1, P2, P3 and P4 to reflect progressively more elaborate containment were described. Roughly speaking, P1 facilities represented stringent, commonsense cleanliness; P2 laboratories had features in common with a surgical operating theatre; P3 containment resembled a giant germ-free isolator and P4 units outdid the most stringent biological warfare establishments. Finally, certain experiments involving highly pathogenic microbes were banned altogether, despite the overall lifting of the moratorium. Later actions by the Director of the National Institutes of Health set up a detailed code of laboratory practice, along the general lines recommended by Asilomar, but buttressed by much greater detail, and significantly stricter.

Lifting the Moratorium unleashes Opposing Views

Perhaps predictably, the scientists who supported the original Berg letter did not receive much praise from society for their openness and caution; but the much larger group that lifted the moratorium certainly faced bitter opposition from lay groups and from a small but significant number of leading scientists. Despite the eloquent pleas of authorities like Nobel Laureate Joshua Lederberg, who referred to the certain and enormous promise of genetic engineering, and the entirely conjectural nature of the risks, the prophets of doom received the lion's share of the publicity. Noted microbiologist Robert Sinsheimer urged a continuation of the pause, because of what he referred to as the potential for biological havoc that the novel forms of rapidly-dividing organisms could wreak. He also raised profound sociological questions: 'How far will we want to develop genetic engineering? Do we want to assume the basic responsibility for life on this planet—to develop new living forms for our own purpose? Shall we take into our own hands our own future evolution?' Erwin Chargaff, an early pioneer in DNA research, urged a delay in further research, if necessary of two or three years, till some host other than E. coli, perhaps a marine organism, could be found.

The most direct confrontation between scientists and the lay public occurred in 1976, in that Mecca of pure science, Cambridge, Massachusetts, the home of both Harvard University and The Massachusetts Institute of Technology. The trigger point was a proposal to build a P3 laboratory. Opponents of recombinant DNA research, including some very prominent scientists, raised the matter with the City Council, which took the unprecedented step of imposing its own three-month moratorium on genetic engineering, a move apparently seen as legal within Harvard and M.I.T. The end result was a local Review Board which set its own safety and health standards, over and above those of the National Institutes of Health.

The idea of local councils buying into the debate did not spread. The United States and United Kingdom examples of containment guidelines enforced largely by peer group pressure (and grant cuts for transgressions) were taken up in many countries, including Australia. On the whole, this system appears to have worked well, with only one or two examples of failure to comply having come to notice. Detailed and far-reaching legislation was, indeed, seriously considered in the United States, but not proceeded with. This pattern was repeated in several European countries.

The Genie turns out to be Benign

In the event, none of the fears of the prophets of doom materialized. The capacity of E. coli K12, the strain most commonly used as a host for recombined vectors, to establish itself in the human gut was shown to be quite limited. Individuals fed massive doses of this strain excreted a few viable organisms in their faeces for a few days, then the E. coli disappeared. In fact, this is not surprising, because the whole history of microbiology suggests that when bacteria are grown repeatedly and for long periods on artificial media, they progressively lose the capacity to infect the original host. Furthermore, microbiological containment really does work and even were it imperfect, there is an immense difference between swallowing a billion E. coli intentionally, and ingesting one or ten organisms accidentally. The experience of literally thousands of laboratories now engaged in recombinant DNA research has proved that the technology as such is entirely safe, and not a single health incident has been reported since the moratorium was lifted. Of course, the spectre of someone using the technology for evil purposes, such as germ warfare, cannot be discounted. All one can say is that no evidence of this type of research has surfaced. With the benefit of hindsight, it is now possible to state that none of the conjectural hazards materialized, and that the initial containment guidelines were unnecessarily stringent. Indeed, in early 1979, the National Institutes of Health relaxed the levels of containment somewhat, many experiments edging down one level, e.g. from requirement for a P3 laboratory to P2, etc. Most other countries followed suit. I confidently expect this process to continue, and believe that the great majority of recombinant DNA work will eventually require little more than commonsense cleanliness in the laboratory, that is, P1 facilities.

Another success story has been the apparent world-wide voluntary compliance of industry with the guidelines in each country. This is admirable, as submitting research protocols to monitoring committees must have occasionally involved revelations of corporate strategy normally kept secret for commercial reasons.

Opposition to Genetic Engineering in a Historical Setting

Now that the illusory fears can be put to one side, we can approach the questions posed at the beginning of this chapter with more realism. It is a fact that this technology, and extensions of it which can be logically foreseen, give mankind the possibility to find out more about the basic processes of life than ever before, and to create life forms in ways that nature never intended. These vast new powers frighten many people.

In fact, there is nothing new about a distrust of science. In his brilliant essay, 'Reflections on the Neo-Romantic Critique of Science', Leo Marx reminds us that many of the eighteenth-century writers questioned 'the legitimacy of science both as a mode of cognition and as a social institution'. Alfred North Whitehead saw this romantic reaction as 'a protest on behalf of the organic view of nature, and also a protest against the exclusion of value' from the sober array of facts which are the fruits of scientific work. Somehow, the Arcadian vision of nature as good, supreme, bountiful, was challenged by the impersonal machines of technology that were eroding nature's grip on human destiny. While the reliability of scientific knowledge within its own frame of reference has really not been seriously questioned since the days of Galileo, Whitehead sees a discrepancy between what science provides in the way of knowledge, and what mankind actually wants by way of a meaningful existence. Strangely, the romantic writers make scant mention of the effects of science and technology on the crushing burdens of work which the poor were forced to assume in order to eke out a meagre existence. More recently, C. P. Snow lamented the gap between the 'two cultures', but even he did not foresee the intensity of the dissident movement, the intelligent anti-science counter-culture, which reached its crescendo in the Vietnam war era. This saw science as the villain responsible not only for the tools of destruction but for fostering a mentality that could allow them to be used.

Basically, the opposition to major technological change, and thus indirectly to science, comes in two forms. On the one hand, there is a tendency for people to fear the unknown, to resist change, to preserve comfortable preconceptions, to resent new circumstances not of their own making. This kind of objection is best countered by modulating the rate of technological change, and while this is a major challenge for politicians and other decision-makers, the body politic has the capacity at least to address the issue and make appropriate choices.

The second class of objection is more difficult to counter. It is more abstract, and relates to whether a scientific view of nature, after all a rather recent event in human affairs, some-how robs mankind of other ways of finding truth or knowledge. Theodore Roszak wonders whether an ingrained commitment to science as the reality principle 'frustrates our best efforts to achieve wholeness'. He links mankind's recent flirtation with science and technology to the sometimes terrifying trend to urbanization, and deplores the 'technocratic elitism' which characterizes not only the industrialized countries but also dominates the leadership of most developing countries.

It would be altogether too facile to dismiss this category of opposition to science as being Luddite responses of disaffected minorities. Many able and intelligent people perceive a genuine threat. For example, Pope John Paul II, in an address to UNESCO, expressed the following view:

> The future of man and mankind is threatened, radically threatened, in spite of very noble intentions, by men of science ... their discoveries have been and continue to be exploited—to the prejudice of ethical imperatives—to ends ... of destruction and death to a degree never before attained, causing unimaginable ravages ... This can be verified as well in the realm of genetic manipulations and biological experiments as well as in those of chemical, bacteriological or nuclear armaments.

This might appear an extreme view, but we must ask why the various counter-cultures, having in common a rejection of popular material and economic goals, enjoy so much support. Furthermore, a decline in participation in the 'harder' natural sciences has been noted in schools, as well as an increased interest in the 'softer' social sciences. So disillusionment with science and technology runs deep in some segments of society.

In Defence of Scientific Truth

This vision of science as somehow anti-human, coldly perverting people from a truly satisfying destiny, must be refuted, because it offends common sense—it is simply not true. If fault there be, it lies in mankind's nature and the uses to which power may be put.

Science and technology have been embraced by people all over the world for one simple reason: they work. Sir Peter Medawar has argued that 'science, broadly considered, is incomparably the most successful enterprise human beings have ever engaged upon'. We do not have to go all the way with Marcelin Berthelot who declared that science 'will provide the truly human basis of morals and politics in the future'. Nevertheless, it is unfair to blame science and technology for ills in the human condition that are as old as mankind: for undue aggression, selfishness, greed and a chronic incapacity to live up to one's highest aspirations. It is as illogical to blame science and technology for not slaking our thirst for spirituality and transcendence as it would be to blame literature, art and music for not feeding, clothing and sheltering us. Science can only address part of the phenomenon of man. In my experience, few people realize this more fully than the scientists themselves, who, as a group, are better read and more concerned with humanistic values than many other technical and professional groups.

There are undoubtedly some who will say that genetic engineering research offends nature, that the creation of new life forms should be left in the hands of evolution, not in mankind's. We must listen to this view, but also be careful to explain to its proponents that conventional genetic techniques employed by civilizations for ten thousand years have already had a formidable impact on the ecosystem, and it might indeed be difficult to distinguish, say, a disease-resistant strain of wheat created by scientific breeding and selection pre-1975 from one fashioned tomorrow through the new technology. Should we really stop ourselves from accelerating the search for moulds making better or cheaper antibiotics because DNA splicing is somehow intrinsically bad? Well, if it appears that this makes little sense, should we at least declare 'hands off' genetic engineering of higher life forms such as mammals? But if genetic manipulation of growth hormones were to allow a steer to grow to full size in six months rather than three years, is it evil to create such animals given that we already have feed lots, and that the world is hungry for first class protein?

What, then, about human beings as genetic guinea pigs? This is clearly the area that has caused the most concern and also confusion. At the moment, the only realistic possibilities that can be foreseen are manipulations of cells and tissues of a given sick human individual, one of whose genes is unhealthy. This seems worth while and noble if it can be achieved. There is currently no approach which can cure single gene defects inside a person so as to repair the genes in all the sperms or all the ova. Accordingly, the only way of eradicating bad genes (or repairing them) for the benefit of future generations is to contemplate treatment of sperm, ova or early embryos in the test tube, prior to artificial insemination or embryo transplantation. Given that practical ways of doing this may be decades away, and that sperm or ovum selection may be more practical in many situations involving recessive gene traits, there still appears to be nothing that mankind should fear in this approach.

Now we come to the famous 'thin edge of the wedge' style of argument. 'If you are curing thalassaemia today, will you not be tackling social rebelliousness tomorrow? If we allow this kind of thing to start, where will it all stop?' The first defence, but not the most important one, I believe, is that we still have only the sketchiest of notions about the processes of inheritance that govern complex features of character, or even most physical attributes such as strength, beauty, tendency to obesity and so forth. These are clearly the results of the interplay of a multiplicity of genes; and of societal and environmental forces impinging on each individual. They are therefore simply not amenable to gene therapy, and may never be. Even were this not the case, I find myself out of tune with a line of reasoning which says: 'I will not do this good thing, because it might lead me on to do that bad thing'. The whole history of mankind has been to probe, to examine, to explore, to seek the limits of understanding and then to exceed them, each generation building on the legacy of its predecessors. To deny that thirst for knowledge is to destroy mankind's wholeness, more surely than anything else.

And what if the chemical nature of man is the object under study? Is it healthy for us to know we are 'just' a few DNA molecules being copied and read? The answer again is blindingly clear. Of course it is good for us to know more about what we are; at worst, this knowledge might allow us to prevent and cure our most obvious ailments; at best, it might even help us to deal more effectively with one another. No knowledge of a natural truth gained by objective search can be harmful, though its misuse obviously can. Furthermore, no depth of insight into the physical nature of man that we can derive from scientific experimentation will detract from or compete with the insights that we gain through the humanities, though indeed a complementation is an eventual possibility.

Just as the decision whether to pursue recombinant DNA research was never really in doubt, but only an uncertainty about timing and order, so the question of whether to apply the technique to man is not in doubt either. It does raise a whole untidy series of issues which must be faced, one by one, and which will surely look rather different when they are no longer hypothetical. How, then, are we to ensure that the genetic engineering revolution is kept on track, as the servant of society; is harnessed towards noble ends; and is developed at a pace that our civilization cannot only bear but actively welcome? These issues of public policy are discussed in the next chapter.

11
Genetic Engineering and Public Policy

Scientists occupy a strange, even difficult, position in our society. On the one hand, they enjoy considerable freedom to pursue their own interests, exercising their creativity unshackled by the daily demands which constrain most workers. On the other hand, they are, in the main, sustained by public funds, so must in the broadest sense be responsive to society's needs. And, most assuredly, scientists are not above the law. Without a doubt, the power of the scientist to dictate mankind's agenda has grown formidably. Do we now need new laws and new public policies to control the scientists?

Existing Levels of Control on Scientific Experimentation

It is important to point out that, quite properly, today's research worker already faces a battery of controls, acting at many levels, some direct and some indirect, which bear on his or her activities on a daily basis. It is worth examining these in some detail. First, each organization performing research has safety rules, a professional safety officer and a safety committee. All research in an institution must conform to standards imposed by these internal elements. It is now frequent to encounter biohazards committees distinct from the traditional safety committees used to worrying more about fire, explosions or toxic chemicals. Secondly, all research has some kind of funding source, and if large governmental agencies are involved, the granting body will usually have an ethics committee and various more specialized committees certifying the safety of given categories of work. This is the chief lever that has been used so far in recombinant DNA research. Thirdly, if research on human subjects is contemplated, it is necessary to obtain both the informed consent of the person, and the approval of an ethics committee of the hospital or university, such committees always having lay members as well as medical specialists. Fourthly, scientists are answerable to the normal administrative controls of institutions, and thus subject to discipline if they embark on a course of action considered outside accepted norms.

More indirect controls have equal force. Peer group pressure is ever-present in science; peer group approval one of the most eagerly-sought rewards. Now that areas such as genetic engineering, foetal research and organ transplantation have been brought so much into the spotlight, the peer group itself, thoroughly indoctrinated with locally-accepted guidelines, will be a monitor of any would-be dissenter. The publication process, also, is an indirect level of control. For example, experiments involving any unnecessary cruelty to animals may be rejected by an editor, as would any manuscript failing to detail safety precautions in potentially risky experiments. The fiscal mechanism also contributes in an indirect way. If a line of work, though not directly contravening a safety rule, nevertheless seems near the borderline, its originator may well find the going a little tougher when a final priority score for funding is assigned.

All the above controls arise, to a greater or lesser degree, from within the scientific enterprise. What of controls from the outside? Again, in some areas such as permissible levels of radiation or toxic wastes, there are specific regulations and laws imposed at federal, state or local levels. Genetic engineering has so far largely avoided this level of control. However, there is also the precious heritage of the common law. If a recombinant DNA research group were to flout the safety standards, regulations and guidelines accepted in a particular country, and some harm were to come to one or more individuals, the injured party could sue, and would probably win. One of the surest proofs of the safety of genetic engineering research carried on to date is that this has not yet happened!

Specific Legislation or Flexible Guidelines?

This set of answers does not satisfy those critics of science who believe that the public should have more say in what scientists do, or are allowed to do. The critics argue for specific legislation covering areas deemed controversial or risky. Such legislation has been in force for years in the field of organ transplantation, and appears to have been well accepted by both patients and doctors. Legislation also covers foetal research and areas such as artificial insemination, in vitro fertilization and induced abortion in most countries. This has resulted in a great deal of controversy, bitterness and even hatred. In some instances, widespread flouting of the law has occurred. Are new laws the answer to better development of genetic engineering?

Proponents of specific legislation make a number of cogent points for their case. Microbiological agents such as disease-causing organisms are clearly dangerous and are already covered by various laws and regulations. Should not the new potential for creating still more dangerous variants be covered by extensions or amendments to these laws? Moreover, if a technology has the potential to cause catastrophic damage (e.g. release into the environment of an extraordinarily toxic engineered microbe; or uncontrolled weed-like spread of some plant variety with superior growth characteristics), might a point be reached where society should seek protection under the law rather than relying on voluntary restraints? Laws might also ensure that monitoring committees would include a full spectrum of community views, and would have real powers. Furthermore, an indirect argument holds that many of the implications of rapid scientific development are not being addressed sufficiently by lawmakers; perhaps the dramatic example of genetic engineering could serve as a triggering point to alert the legal profession and the politicians to their responsi-bilities. Finally, a call for new legislation might be one factor encouraging greater public participation in the debate about where science is taking the world. All these views require care-ful examination.

Having followed this debate closely for a decade, and having developed great respect for some of the able proponents of an opposite viewpoint, my conclusion is against the introduction of new laws on genetic engineering. I see many complexities and no advantages in going down the legislative route in this field. First, the technology is changing so rapidly that legislation would be extremely difficult to draft; the boundaries of genetic engineering are constantly being extended and the distinction between it and the rest of cellular and molecular biology are becoming blurred. For example, *infusing* DNA from one cell into another would be classified as genetic engineering, but *fusing* the two living cells to achieve genetic hybridization would not. Legislation would probably require amendment before the printer's ink were dry. Secondly, society's worst nightmares know no geographic boundaries, but laws do. If a particular nation were to enact restrictive legislation in the recombinant DNA field today, this would not stop the research;

it would simply move it to another country. There are instances of this happening; for example, where one country demanded P4 level of containment, the most rigorous and expensive laboratory facility, for an experiment which another classified as P3, a substantially less elaborate set-up. The only end-result of a given country taking a 'tough line' with its scientists would be that the country would simply hand the lead in the forbidden area to countries with a different viewpoint. Thirdly, the passage of legislation would still not offer the critics what they want; namely, control of issues by non-scientists. Much of the legislation would have to be highly technical, and provisional until conjectural hazards were subjected to more testing, so that experts in the field would essentially have to do all the drafting and make all the tough decisions. This comes back more or less to the present position! Fourthly, the horror situations that have been painted lack realism. It is very doubtful whether it would be possible to tailor-make plant varieties that truly spread like wildfire, or to invent germs more horrible than the ones, like Lassa fever or botulism, that we already possess. Finally, it is important to recall that none of the conjectural hazards that have been mooted have in fact materialized.

Rather than legislation, I prefer the soft-edged, untidy, polyvalent methods of a free and decent society. I believe in a fundamental residue of idealism within the biomedical research community. I believe the threshold of consciousness about risks has been raised to the extent that most silly things will be stopped before they happen. I believe both scientists and the regulators have gained much from nearly a decade's intensive debate. I think the fundamental challenge now is not to control but to promote recombinant DNA research.

Biological Species as Intellectual Property

Before leaving the legal arena, it is worth noting that in 1980, by the slimmest possible majority of 5 to 4, the Supreme Court of the United States decreed that a living organism could constitute a patentable entity. This opened the way for commercial enterprises to increase their involvement in genetic engineering under the same kind of patent protection as applies, for example, to drugs or chemicals. It also legitimized a patent that Stanley Cohen and Herbert Boyer had taken out covering the broad technology used in most genetic engineering work. This means that Stanford University and the University of California at San Francisco will get licence fees and royalties from essentially all products of genetic engineering that reach the market, unless the patent is challenged. Only time will tell whether this represents a mammoth income for the two universities.

Obviously, the patenting of living organisms raises some tough legal issues, far beyond the scope of a book such as the present one. The interested reader is referred to a fine work sponsored by the Cold Spring Harbor Laboratory entitled *Patenting of Life Forms*, edited by David W. Plant and others, which collects the views of both interested scientists and some of the most distinguished jurists working in the field.

An unusual suggestion that has recently come forward is that copyright laws might apply to genetically engineered microbes or tissue-cultured cells. Dr Irving Kayton, Professor of Law at The George Washington University, argues that in the United States, the Copyright Act offers an effective and desirable way of protecting the commercial interests of genetic and cellular engineers, perhaps giving greater protection than patents or practices of commercial secrecy. He makes analogies between gene libraries and computer programmes, each being a compilation resembling an original work of authorship. Copyright protection lasts much longer than patent protection, namely from the time of creation to fifty years after the death of the author, as compared with seventeen to twenty-seven years from invention for patents. This concept has only recently entered the arena and has not yet been tested in the courts.

The Need for Increased Communication between Science, Industry and Government

In Chapter 9 we noted that various governments are actively promoting components of the DNA industry in their countries. In view of the storm that surrounded the birth of genetic engineering, and the enduring concern for more regulations and legislation in some quarters, should more be done to keep politicians and jurists abreast of this field? What can we do as a society to make decision-makers at many levels of society more aware of this and other issues involving high technology and scientific specialization?

In my opinion, this issue is currently far more important than the one of new legislation. To address it, we must first ask why a need for more extensive communication and debate exists. The central difficulty is the ignorance—and indeed apathy—within the community about the research process and about the nexus between fundamental research and applied development. Our lives are affected by technological change at a daily level and in the most diverse ways. The future will bring further technological changes. Some of these we hope for fervently (a cure for cancer; pollution-free vehicles) and others we antici-pate with a mixture of admiration and apprehension (more robots in factories; rocket-powered travel). In either case, the vast majority of us are concerned exclusively with the practical end-result of scientific development; with the completed exper-iments that impinge directly on our lives. But all these changes, from the most important to the most trivial, depend on people; on scientists and technologists manning the formidable enter-prise of global research and development. Almost by definition, these people are specialists. They live within a linked spectrum of subcultures, and, in general, exercise their influence within the world of ideas rather than through the acknowledged realms of power, namely politics or business. Thus, there are very few scientists in the world's parliaments or, with some exceptions, in leadership positions within public service. Per-haps more surprisingly, there are few scientists in management positions within industry or commerce, even in high technology industries. So the people with the technical capacity to shape the future are under-represented within the highest levels of decision-making.

Scientists and technologists know full well the dynamic inter-play between curiosity-motivated basic probing of concepts and mission-oriented study of some hoped-for practical advance. In general, they know what can be anticipated with near-certainty provided enough effort is expended; what rep-resents a fair gamble for the medium term; and what is still beyond reach. They know further that the only hope of bringing the last category of advances to eventual fruition is by sustain-ing a broadly-based, patient effort in fundamental research aimed simply at understanding nature in all its manifold mani-festations. But the general public knows little about this, and, worse still, cares little.

This separation of the process of research and technological change from the process of leadership and governance of society imposes the need for better communication. It should be a communication between equals, pursued with objectivity and neutrality. The scientists should inform the public about what they are doing; about what practical results can realisti-cally be expected; and about what longer-term dreams can legi-timately be espoused. Society, through all the means of com-munication and leverage available, should respond and thereby guide the science enterprise into those broad subject areas requiring most emphasis. This process is, of course, going on in most countries, but labours under certain constraints.

Structural Problems impeding Objective Communication

The first constraint relates to the knowledge base within society. Most people, including many influential leaders, lack the patience and the intellectual stamina to follow scientific arguments, even if these are structured in simple, non-technical language. In many respects, though so deeply influenced by the end-results of science, we are a scientifically illiterate society. As one who has struggled hard to make modern biology accessible to lay audiences of diverse types, I am only too familiar with the glazed look or patent discomfiture that is the frequent reward for my efforts! Some mental trapdoor seems to evoke memories of schoolroom tortures, defences spring up which say: 'this is intended for someone really clever; I'd better leave it all to the experts'. The simplest response for the scientist is to get to the 'bottom line'—the practical implications of the research—very quickly, thereby losing much of the story.

The scientist, too, bears much of the blame for suboptimal communication. Two deficiencies are particularly common. First, the scientist either will not or cannot make the adjustments required to alter the mode of communication from a technical to a popular one. One of the cardinal sins in a scientific paper is to make exaggerated claims for the generality of a particular discovery, or to omit the limitations of the scientific approach used, which may require qualification of the general conclusion. Therefore, scientific papers use a contrived, stylized, rather coy prose form full of phrases like: 'Table III appears to indicate that . . .'; 'the results are consistent with the following interpretation . . .'; 'within the limitations of the present experimental design . . .'; etc. Furthermore, the paper will usually be full of technical terms that seem quite commonplace to the investigator, so much so that their obscurity to the layman occasions surprise. When discoveries are translated for popular consumption, it is better to go to the heart of the matter and omit the minor qualifications, provided that the listener or reader is not left with an inflated idea of what has happened. It is also necessary to use familiar terms and perhaps homely analogies to get the message across. Secondly, scientists find it hard to be objective and neutral about their own work, and often foray into the realms of communication with the layman only when they want something—usually a larger grant! This, obviously, creates a predictable reaction. Decision-makers discount the scientist's claim, sometimes appropriately, but frequently to a more than necessary extent. Too much of the communication takes place in a setting that has at least a component of an adversary relationship; too little in the context of free brainstorming out of sheer interest.

These constraints show up most clearly in the area of pure or fundamental research. I firmly believe an innate scepticism about its value limits the commitment which politicians are willing to make to universities and similar institutions. Again, this is not all the fault of the politicians. The message that giant strides in mankind's capacity to control nature result from the most unlikely, curiosity-motivated research cannot be repeated too frequently. Who would have predicted that research on some obscure bacterial enzyme which can chop up DNA into little bits would sponsor a new industrial revolution? Analysis of all the major developments in technology soon reveal their dependence on prior basic research, and revelation of this nexus should form part of every attempt at popularization of science.

The Role of the Public Sector in promoting Genetic Engineering

The above discussion is critical in tone, but at the same time I believe the situation is improving, and, for the biological sciences, the DNA story has done much to prompt greater efforts at discourse between scientists and the rest of society. The above problems do not lend themselves to easy or definitive solution. They require gradual attitudinal changes and steady effort. Indeed, this book itself is one small example of what can be done to break down the barrier in communication, an effort made easier by society's lively interest in anything that affects health. It may be a presumptuous conclusion, but I sense that society is now ready for the public sector to take an active role in the promotion of genetic engineering, in part because of the serious work that has been done from both sides of the fence.

There are three levels at which public policy can have a major effect. Each has been creatively attacked through recent initiatives in Australia, but the principles involved are general ones applicable to all countries. The first level involves the creation of a cadre of scientists and technologists capable of participating in the DNA industry at a high level of expertise.

While excellent undergraduate courses are obviously necessary, they are not sufficient. The most cost-effective way of enlarging the pool of trained workers is to encourage an expansion of the research teams of established leaders in the field. This should be through a peer-group-reviewed research grant mechanism, but one with guidelines that make it clear that projects to be sponsored should have a substantial component of applied science. Such a mechanism has a built-in quality control device, and also a relatively short lag period, giving it advantages over more elaborately structured and expensive national educational plans.

The second level involves the encouragement of venture capital formation, preferably in a manner that makes large as well as small enterprises look closely at the risk-reward equation in this field. Tax incentives represent one simple and effective way of doing this; long-term, low interest loans another; and equity participation by governmental bodies a third. In smaller countries, access to capital alone may not be sufficient to establish a biotechnology industry. Mechanisms that help inventors or entrepreneurs gain access to managerial expertise may be important. To help the small firms to develop a discovery, government departments may have to provide advice on markets, feasibility, international trade potential, and so forth. Export incentives will be especially valuable for countries with a limited domestic consumer market. A supportive stance by government in the early years is probably necessary in most countries if they are to have any chance of competing with the United States in this field.

A third area to which attention must be given is the relationship between academic departments advancing DNA research and industrial concerns anxious to exploit these advances. This remark may seem trite, but it is curious how substantial a gap still separates these two universes of endeavour, despite the rapprochement mentioned in Chapter 9. In addition to the spontaneous developments mentioned there, specific government policies can narrow the gap by mechanisms which tempt the academic to seek out a commercial partner more actively. For example, a scheme recently introduced in Australia gives grants preferentially to academic departments which have formed formal linkages with firms willing and able to take the resulting discoveries to the stage of commercialization. Schemes which promote interchange of workers between universities, institutes and industry also have appeal. These could encourage younger scientists to cross the barriers for seconded periods of two to three years, and could provide for sabbatical periods of six to twelve months for senior workers. It would be important to have traffic in both directions and to safeguard the career prospects of the participants. Such schemes cost little, but create a climate where the traditional distrust would be broken down quite rapidly, given a society where each of the two sectors is doing its job properly.

Obviously, detailed patterns of government intervention would vary in each nation, and over time. It is pleasing to record that public policy in Australia is moving in precisely these directions. Australia is a country with a small population, and not noted for the success of its manufacturing industry. There is an urgent requirement for the manufacturing sector to become more competitive in world terms. A tradition of excellence in biological research at the basic level, and a broad recognition that biotechnology offers opportunities for the creation of high value products where the distance from export markets is not such a drastic disadvantage, presage an exciting future in the decade ahead.

12
Distant Horizons

Speculations about the future of genetic engineering tend to fall into three groups, each possessing able and vocal proponents. There are those most excited about the industrial and commercial potential, who see new Silicon Valleys emerging, capable of jetting whole nations into a new golden age of prosperity. Then there are those whose dominant concern is with twin dangers. They fear a wilful or accidental release of highly pathogenic species into the biosphere. They also worry that an excessively mechanistic appreciation of the nature of life may further drive mankind towards materialism and a sterile, stereotyped view of the universe, devoid of subtlety or value. Finally there are the scientists themselves, many of whom believe that molecular biology is the new key to the solution of essentially all the deep puzzles still confronting them, and therefore the discipline beyond all others requiring emphasis and support.

The realities are, of course, much more complex than that, and each extreme requires comment. The fact that a process or product is labelled 'genetic engineering' or 'high technology', for that matter, does not endow it with magical properties that permit it instantly to overwhelm the marketplace and make its sponsors wealthy. In each of the industrial applications we have discussed, genetically engineered products will have to prove their superiority, one by one, over presently-available alternatives. This will undoubtedly be a tough battle, in which there will be a few winners and many losers. Observers of Silicon Valley rarely point out that for every successful Californian electronics company, there were literally scores of failures, and there is no reason to believe that it will be any different for the DNA industry. While the widespread publicity about genetic engineering has achieved a highly worthwhile raising of public consciousness about commercial possibilities, the important thing for the immediate and more distant future will be to engage in meticulous and realistic case-by-case analysis of opportunities against a background of justifiable long-term optimism.

The Dangers foreseen from Genetic Engineering will continue to prove Groundless

Neither of the sets of dangers foreseen for genetic engineering will materialize. As regards ecological or epidemic disaster situations, we have already covered the efficacy of existing safeguards in Chapters 10 and 11, and here I wish to make a further speculative point. Evolution has had a very long time to create the present, constantly changing but nevertheless balanced and extraordinarily diverse biological landscape of this planet. It has done so by ensuring that DNA can change down the generations. Copying errors can be made, changing individual genes. New genes can be introduced into cells from the outside by viruses or other vectors. Genes can jump around within a cell. Genes are constantly being placed into novel constellations through the processes of sexual reproduction. This has sometimes given us species that startle us with their capacity to cause havoc, such as the bacteria of bubonic plague, or the grasshopper devastating whole tracts of crops. Yet even the worst examples of what evolution can do to place the ecosystem at the mercy of a single species reach their limits in space and in time. The plague did not destroy Western civilization. The grasshopper did not put an end to planned agriculture. While not doubting the capacity of genetic engineering to come up with species with quite amazing qualities, I cast doubt upon the capacity of any such species totally to wreck the world. The feedback loops within the ecosystem are too many and varied for that to happen. There is only one species that can wreck the world, and that is man himself, with the nuclear weapons he has invented.

This brings us to the second set of alleged dangers. I argued in Chapter 10 that scientific results and insights were not dehumanizing, but rather energized much of what is best in mankind. Here I want to go one step further, to suggest that a fuller understanding of man's biological nature, not by a few experts, but by large masses of people, could prove to be a very liberating influence. Ignorance, superstition, fear of unknowable dark forces, oppression by the few gifted with knowledge and power—these have been the impediments which over the centuries have fettered the human spirit. A conviction that even the most profound and obscure realities—the nature of consciousness, the uniqueness of each individual—are the results of orderly processes, which obey rules and possess structure, must allow a person to confront his or her destiny with a heightened awareness and strength. If, further to that, a belief grows that these rules and structures are knowable, this surely permits man to walk into the future tall and free-striding, more determined to shape that future himself. As the biological basis of the phenomenon of man is gradually revealed, I have no doubt that, far from leading to a sterile or uniform vision, a richly-patterned, fine-grained mosaic will emerge, dazzling in its complexity, diversity and subtlety. We are a long way from that point, groping about as we are at this taxonomic and descriptive stage of gene research. We cannot yet pick Einstein from a dullard or Mozart from a tone-deaf philistine on the basis of DNA sequence data. But we have made a beginning. We can describe the differences between the genetic make-up of two people more fully than ever before. We can say profound things about the diseases each is more likely to get, and the biochemical weaknesses each is capable of passing down to offspring. Of necessity, our first concern has been with abnormalities, potentially capable of detection, but analysis of variances between normal people, as a problem in its own right, has also begun. The correlation of these with those physical or mental characteristics that matter to us will be an awesome task, the work of centuries rather than decades, but we need certainly not fear what the search will uncover.

Genetic engineering has revealed the universality, beauty and order of the rules of biology. These rules create the diversity of life that we revere and cherish. It now appears a matter of prime importance that the central truths which are emerging find their way into the school curricula, not only for that small proportion of children and youths who choose to study biology as a specialty, but indeed for all future citizens. In the deepest sense, DNA's structure and function have become as much part of our cultural heritage as Shakespeare, the sweep of history, or any of the things we expect an educated person to know. The era in which the fundamentals of molecular biology and genetic engineering are taught in high school could well prove to be the era when man finally becomes comfortable with science, one of his prize creations, and more mature in ensuring that its power is harnessed towards noble ends.

Molecular Biology the King of the Biosciences?

The third set of futurologists, coming from within science, tend not to air their speculations within public fora, but rather to exert influence within the system in an unarticulated but nevertheless effective way. I speak of the decision-makers, the trend-setters and the role models leading science from within the academic community. There is the widespread assumption that molecular biology has won pride of place as the most important discipline within science. To be a molecular biologist is best of all; if you are some other kind of biologist, you had better find yourself a molecular biologist as a collaborator, or you will be left behind in the race. Molecular biology is to be valued above all because it is the great harmonizing and welding force in biology that unifies all the specialties; and, of course, genetic engineering is the key tool of the molecular biologist.

There is much of merit in such an analysis, but also much to doubt and a little to fear. Let there be no question about the critical role which molecular biology and genetics are playing as tools in the great adventure of contemporary bioscience. Whether you are in medicine, veterinary science or agriculture; whether you seek pure biological knowledge or some practical goal; whether your specialty involves the brain or the liver or the immune system; the problem you are addressing will at some level involve cells and the intricate communication between cells. These processes involve protein molecules; understanding them means understanding protein structure; interfering with them for good or ill means introducing drugs or other interventions which mimic or impede specific proteins. Genetic engineering, because of the superior technologies invented over the last decade, gives us the power to study DNA, RNA and protein structure in an entirely new way and with breathtaking speed. It has superseded many other ways of approaching biological problems, and immensely complemented many others. If there is any prediction about more distant horizons which I can make with complete certainty, it is that genetic engineering will yield basic information about diverse biological systems which will more than justify the resources devoted to it. Perhaps its contribution to fundamental research will prove to be its main gift.

Even though scientific research is changing, and its technologic complexity is increasing phenomenally, I still believe research is principally about ideas. Advanced techniques are absolutely essential tools, and the prizes in science may well chiefly fall to those hands that master the most tools, or deploy them most effectively; but the logical and imaginative constructs that human minds produce when the tools have done their work are the essence of science, and that which distinguishes it from technology (or research from development). It is therefore important to remember that genetic engineering is a tool. In biology, as I am sure, in physical sciences, the complex real-life situations which we seek to comprehend can be viewed from many perspectives. Let us take a simple example from medicine, say a patient with multiple sclerosis. The neurologist will look at this as a problem in diagnosis and therapy; the perspective will be analysis of symptoms, signs and diagnostic tests. Given the uniqueness of that particular patient's case, one or other remedy of an available set will be chosen. The clinical immunologist, on the other hand, is more conerned with causative mechanisms: is the disease due to a virus gone underground, or to an inappropriate immune attack or both? He, then, turns to any one of a number of neuroscientist colleagues. One will investigate in detail the impaired nerve conduction, using complex electronic recording apparatus. Another will study antibodies present in the patient's serum, to see if some capable of damaging nerves are present. A third will look to see if the patient has certain genes known to increase the risk; a fourth will be more concerned to determine in detail what molecules on the nerve have been attacked by the ravages of disease. But beyond the neurologist and the neuroscientist, 'above' and 'below' them, if we may caricaturize it, stand others involved in the study of the multiple sclerosis problem. 'Above' we find the epidemiologist trying to make sense of the peculiar geographic distribution of the disease, and the expert in community medicine working out how best to look after the patients, given the limited resources available. 'Below' we have the full spectrum of fundamental biosciences, as these may impinge on brain structure, organization and function.

The point of this simple example is that each of the relevant perspectives is a valid and valuable one. Within each frame of reference, new knowledge will accrue, new insights will enhance capacity to intervene and finally, one day, the puzzle will be solved and the human energies thus released will attack other problems. Each of the levels of search and striving, while seeking all manner of ways to communicate with the level immediately 'up' or 'down' from it, will preserve its own idiom and its own disciplinary integrity; and each one will reserve a special place for the new problems posed as each solution comes to hand. For this multidimensional network which is world science, I see nothing but limitless growth into the indefinite future. If this is so, it is also important to preserve balance and order between the disciplinary layers. It would make no more sense to plough all new resources in the multiple sclerosis field into epidemiology than it would into immunology or electro-physiological diagnostic equipment.

The trick, therefore, for world biological science will be to exploit the truly wondrous potential of genetic engineering without doing harm to other fertile disciplines. Many of the exciting problems on which genetic engineers work stem from within their own framework, but many more come from the outside. Cancer biologists, immunologists, endocrinologists, neurobiologists and many others are crying out for collegial assistance from genetic engineers, so much so that there is a slight danger of transmitting to the younger generation the signal that this is the only way to go. Yet, most of the phenomena for which we seek molecular explanations will continue to come from outside sources, and we need scientists committed to (and steeped in the folklore of) the 'higher' disciplines to provide a continuing stream of cannon-fodder for the genetic engineers.

Why do I term an exaggerated commitment to genetic engineering only a slight danger? Because, all in all, I believe the world science system to be in fine condition, full of all manner of self-correcting mechanisms. That is not to say it could not be improved. We hear much about the fierce competition for grant funds, particularly among younger research workers not yet established in a career structure. Scientists are apprehensive about new intrusions by industry, dissatisfied by treatment in the media, worried about over-regulation, always scornful of politicians' lack of understanding. Yet, beyond all that, there is an excitement and an elation that is barely containable. Biology is in the midst of an explosive leap, one which will make decades of work for future historians. 1984 is a poor year for Orwellian soothsayers. It is a great time to be young in biomedical science.

Suggestions for Further Reading

The following books have been listed in ascending order of difficulty. It is recommended that you begin at the top and work down!

Judson, H. F. (1979) *The Eighth Day of Creation* (Simon & Schuster, New York), 686 pp.

This book is highly recommended as a first class piece of scientific journalism. The author spent seven years researching the saga of DNA, and has interviewed most of the key figures who have created the molecular biology revolution. The book is a mixture of popular science, recent history and material of considerable human interest. Parts of it are far from easy, but a little skipping here and there would not destroy the narrative flow. The book ends where the genetic engineering explosion is about to begin.

Watson, J. D. and Tooze, J. (1981) *The DNA Story* (W. H. Freeman & Co., San Francisco), 605 pp.

This fascinating work describes the unfolding story of genetic engineering by reproducing a large number of primary documents, including press articles, private correspondence, meeting reports, congressional testimony and draft legislation. The authors have annotated the material with short essays which introduce each section, and have provided a brief, beautifully illustrated description of recombinant DNA technology.

Cherfas, J. (1982) *Man Made Life* (Basil Blackwell, Oxford), 270 pp.

This book covers much of the same ground as my present effort, but in considerably greater depth and scientific detail. It is much more extensively illustrated, and goes to commendable effort to ascribe scientific credit correctly to the various pioneers in this field. Though the language is much more racy than that of the conventional text book, the work places fairly heavy demands on the reader and is probably more suitable for a person with a university background in physics, chemistry or biology than for a lay reader.

Stryer, L. (1981) *Biochemistry* (2nd ed.) (W. H. Freeman & Co., San Francisco), 949 pp.

This is undoubtedly the best general textbook of biochemistry available for the beginning student in this field. The illustrations (usually several per page) are quite the best I have come across, and the text is brief and pithy. The work is therefore ideal for students who want to place recombinant DNA technology within the broader framework of general biochemistry.

Morison, R. C. and others (1978) *Limits of Scientific Inquiry* Daedalus, Journal of the American Academy of Arts and Sciences, vol. 107, no 2. 240 pp.

This excellent series of essays is not exclusively concerned with genetic engineering, but approaches the wider questions of societal concerns about science, attempts to control research, the importance of scientific freedom and public risk as an issue.

Plant, D. W., Reimers, N. and Zinder, N. D., eds (1982) *Patenting of Life Forms* (Banbury Report 10), Cold Spring Harbor Laboratory, 337 pp.

This book summarizes a conference which brought together leading lawyers and scientists interested not only in the specific subject of the title, but in broader issues of technology and the law. It forms a good starting point for readers with a special interest in the legal aspects of genetic engineering.

In a field that is moving so rapidly, interested readers who wish to keep up with the broad trends would do well to follow *Scientific American* and *The New Scientist*, both highly respected publications, which frequently feature key aspects of molecular biology among their articles.

Glossary

adenine
> One of the small molecular building blocks, called bases, which make up the coding units of DNA and RNA. Often abbreviated to A. In DNA, pairs with thymine (T).

adenosine diphosphate (ADP)
> A molecule consisting of adenine plus a sugar plus two phosphate groups important in the energy economy of a cell. Oxidation of fuel molecules such as glucose permits ADP to take up an extra phosphate and thereby to trap energy.

adenosine triphosphate (ATP)
> A molecule consisting of adenine plus a sugar plus three phosphate groups which acts as the universal currency of free energy in biological systems. Conversion of ATP to ADP releases energy which drives the work of the cell.

adjuvant
> A substance which increases the efficacy of a vaccine, i.e. stimulates the immune response.

AIDS
> A disease, the acquired immune deficiency syndrome, in which certain T lymphocytes are destroyed and the patient is left defenceless against infections.

allosteric effect
> A protein molecule is caused to change shape through union with another molecule. As a result, a new active site is exposed.

amino acid
> Building block of proteins. There are twenty naturally occurring amino acids.

antibody

A special protein molecule made by the immune system of vertebrate animals, specifically tailored to fit other molecules, for example bacterial toxins, much as a given key fits a particular lock.

antigen

A generic term for a molecule with which an antibody reacts.

autoimmune disease

A disease in which the body manufactures antibodies against some component of itself; thus a form of civil warfare in the body, one cell attacking another.

cDNA

A stretch of DNA synthesized by enzymes as a faithful copy of a particular stretch of RNA, which thus preserves the information content of that RNA.

cell

A fundamental organizational unit of all living matter. The simplest forms of life consist of just one cell, e.g. bacteria, algae or certain parasites. Higher life forms are multicellular organisms, permitting specialization of cellular function, i.e. a division of labour between cells.

cell membrane

The fatty outer skin of a cell which separates it from the next cell, from the fluid bathing cells, or from the environment.

cell membrane receptors

Protein molecules, frequently with some sugars attached, which reside in the cell membrane and possess the capacity to bind specifically some molecule which floats past, e.g. a hormone, a nutrient, or a trigger for cellular activation.

chain

Used in the context of a chain of amino acids which follow a sequence determined by the gene for that chain; many proteins consist of two or more chains linked together chemically. Thus insulin has an α and a β chain; many antibody molecules have four chains, two smaller ones called light, and two larger ones called heavy. Usually accompanied by the adjectival noun polypeptide (q.v.) meaning many amino acids.

chromosome

A very long double-stranded DNA molecule packed together with certain proteins which forms a sausage-like entity readily visualized under the microscope when a cell divides. The number of chromosomes per cell is a characteristic of a species; thus man has forty-six chromosomes per cell.

cloning

Causing asexual division. Frequently used as jargon in genetic engineering to describe the sequence of events by which a gene is caused to replicate a large number of times in some foreign host cell.

codon

A sequence of three bases of DNA or RNA which codes for one amino acid.

colony

A clustered group of cells which arose from a single cell by asexual division, thus a bacterial colony may be a visible spot of 1–2 millimetres diameter consisting of millions of bacteria that are growing in a jellified medium.

cosmid

A virus-like vector used by genetic engineers that combines some of the advantages of phages and of plasmids as instruments for the cloning of genes.

cytoplasm

That portion of a cell which is not the nucleus; the site where proteins are made and where chemical energy is generated; the 'factory' portion of the cell.

cytosine

One of the four small molecular building blocks, called bases, which make up the coding units of DNA. Often abbreviated to C. In DNA, C pairs with guanine (G).

differentiation

The process whereby cells gain more specialized function. Thus, as a cell destined to turn into a red blood cell gradually builds up more and more haemoglobin, it is said to differentiate.

diploid

Refers to the number of chromosomes in a cell or a set. Normal cells contain chromosomes in pairs. Thus twenty-three pairs make up the forty-six chromosomes in a normal diploid human cell. Cancer cells are frequently hyper-diploid, i.e. contain more than forty-six chromosomes.

disulphide bond

A chemical linkage between two sulphur-containing amino acids either within a single polypeptide chain or between the component chains of a multichain protein. The disulphide bonds stabilize the shape of a protein and help to keep multichain proteins as a single molecule.

DNA

Deoxyribonucleic acid. A double helical molecule consisting of a sugar-phosphate backbone and a sequence of base pairs constituting the coding units of the genetic code. Particular stretches of DNA constitute a gene, one gene being that stretch which encodes one polypeptide chain.

DNA ligases

Enzymes which catalyse the formation of the chemical bonds needed to weld pieces of DNA together. Thus, DNA ligases may join a gene from an animal cell with DNA from a phage virus, creating recombinant DNA.

E. coli

Escherichia coli. A harmless bacterial species which resides in the human intestine. Frequently used in genetic research, e.g. as a host cell for phages or plasmids carrying recombinant DNA.

electrophoresis

A procedure in which a mixture of molecules is subjected to an electric current ensuring that each molecule moves at a rate influenced by its net electric charge; thus a useful way of analysing and separating complex mixtures of molecules, e.g. proteins.

endonuclease

An enzyme capable of cutting DNA.

endoplasmic reticulum

A system of channels inside the cytoplasm of a cell for the assembly and export of protein molecules.

endotoxin

A molecule derived from the cell wall of bacteria which is highly toxic to animals.

enzyme

A protein molecule capable of catalysing chemical reactions within the body. Enzymes are strategic components of all cellular metabolism.

exon
: That portion of the gene which encodes a portion of the amino acid sequence of the protein. One gene may contain several exons.

expression vectors
: Tools of the genetic engineer which permit a gene to be inserted into a cell in such a manner that, on appropriate signalling, the cell will manufacture large amounts of the protein for which that gene codes.

gel electrophoresis
: A procedure in which a mixture of proteins, nucleic acids or other molecules is made to penetrate into a jellified medium under the influence of a strong electric current. Molecules migrate at a rate dependent on their net electric charge and, on this basis, different molecules can be separated from one another.

gene
: A stretch of DNA containing specific information for the construction of one polypeptide chain or protein. In higher organisms, genes consist of exons and introns, qq.v.

gene activation
: A process in which a command is given which ensures that messenger RNA molecules will be made as copies of the particular gene being activated. Thus, gene activation is the first step in protein synthesis.

genetic code
: The code whereby the structural information for proteins is encoded in the nucleotides of the DNA. Proteins are strings of amino acids, one amino acid out of twenty being chosen for each spot in the string. Nucleic acids are strings of nucleotides, one nucleotide out of a possible four at each spot. A sequence of three nucleotides specifies one amino acid.

genetic engineering
: The technology by which genes can be isolated, transferred to other cells, replicated and activated.

genome
: A noun used to denote the total complement of genes in a cell or individual.

Golgi apparatus
: A packaging centre for the concentration and temporary storage of protein molecules destined for export by the cell.

guanine
>One of the small molecular building blocks, called bases, which make up the coding units of DNA and RNA. Often abbreviated to G. In DNE, paivs with cytosine (C).

haemoglobin
>An iron-containing pigmented protein contained in the red blood cell which is responsible for carrying oxygen around the body and releasing it for the use of the cells.

haemoglobinopathies
>A group of diseases resulting from an abnormality in the gene for one of the chains of haemoglobin.

haemophilia
>A heritable disease in which a protein essential for blood clotting is defective. Patients bleed too readily, particularly after injury.

haploid
>Refers to the number of chromosomes in a cell or set. Most cells contain pairs of chromosomes, known as a diploid set, but the cells for reproduction, the sperms and the ova, contain only half this number, e.g. twenty-three chromosomes in the human, instead of forty-six in other cells. This constitutes a haploid set. The number is restored to forty-six when sperm and egg fuse.

homopolymer tailing
>A procedure by which a string of nucleotides, all the same, is added to the end of one strand of a DNA molecule. This string, e.g. A-A-A-A-A- will readily stick to another DNA molecule tailed with the complementary nucleotides, e.g. T-T-T-T-T.

hormone
>A chemical messenger molecule, travelling in the blood stream, synthesized by cells in an endocrine gland and capable of influencing growth and metabolism within other, perhaps distant, cells which possess receptors for that hormone.

hydrogen bonding
>In a hydrogen bond, a hydrogen atom is shared by two other atoms (in biological systems, nitrogen and oxygen). Hydrogen bonds stabilize the structure of proteins and of DNA.

insulin
>A hormone made by β cells in the pancreas necessary for the proper utilization of glucose within the body.

interferon

A generic term used to describe three groups of molecules, the α β and γ interferons. These molecules are synthesized by cells as a result of virus infection and temporarily interfere with the growth of other viruses in that or nearby cells.

intron

Stretch of DNA occurring within a gene which, however, does not code for amino acids of the relevant protein. When a gene is activated, the RNA molecules made as copies of the gene faithfully reflect both introns and exons (q.v.), but before this RNA travels to the cytoplasm, the sequences corresponding to introns are cut out and the (shorter) RNA corresponding only to copies of exons is joined up to constitute the final messenger RNA template.

lac operon

A group of genes and control elements responsible for the proper utilization of lactose by bacterial cells. Frequently used by genetic engineers as a switching device for gene activation, q.v.

lipase

An enzyme capable of catalysing the digestion of fats.

lipid

A technical term for describing fatty molecules in biology.

lysosomes

Small pouches within the cytoplasm of cells containing enzymes capable of digesting particles or molecules that enter the cell.

major histocompatibility complex

A group of genes which determine the tissue type of an individual, i.e. compatibility with another for organ transplantation. Also involved in the regulation of immune responses.

meiosis

A special type of cell division which creates the reproductive cells, the sperm and the ova. During the process, not only is the number of chromosomes halved, e.g. in the human from forty-six to twenty-three, but also the paternal and maternal genes become recombined in new ways. As this happens differently in each meiotic division, no two sperms or no two ova in any individual are exactly the same.

messenger RNA

A copy of the DNA which moves from nucleus to cytoplasm and

serves as the immediate coding entity which is decoded as proteins are made.

mitochondria
Subcellular particles within the cytoplasm which generate chemical energy for use by the cell in a large number of bioconversions.

mitosis
The non-sexual division of cells whereby each daughter cell receives the full diploid number of chromosomes.

mobile genetic element
Portion of the genome which, unlike most DNA, does not occupy a fixed position but can jump from spot to spot on a chromosome or even move between chromosomes.

molecule
A grouping of atoms which together make a stable substance.

monoclonal antibody
An antibody made by the progeny of a single cell, thus extremely pure, precise and homogeneous.

Niemann-Pick disease
A rare genetic disorder in which a defect in a gene inside the lysosome causes accumulation of lipid inside the cell. Somewhat related to Tay-Sachs disease, q.v.

nucleic acids
Two types of polymer molecules, DNA and RNA (q.v.), which act as the repositories of genetic information. They consist of a backbone of alternating sugar and phosphate portions, with a coding unit attached to each sugar.

nucleotides
The building blocks from which the polymeric nucleic acids are made, i.e. a sugar with an attached coding unit and phosphate group.

nucleus
The control centre of the cell, where the DNA resides, separated from the 'factory' portion of the cell, the cytoplasm, by a double membrane.

oncogene
> A gene or genes which, when inappropriately activated, can be involved in the production of cancer.

organelles
> Small subcellular particulate structures within the cytoplasm of a cell, recognizable in the electron microscope and frequently separable from other organelles or the fluid, structureless part of the cell by biophysical techniques. Many organelles possess specific functions known in detail.

palindromic sequences
> Stretches of DNA which read identically backwards or forwards.

peptide synthesis
> The process by which amino acids are joined together to form short or long chains.

phage
> Abbreviation of bacteriophage virus, a virus capable of infecting and destroying bacteria. Frequently used as a vector (q.v.) by genetic engineers.

phosphorylation
> The metabolic process whereby a phosphate group is added to a molecule.

plaque
> A clear area, e.g. where a phage population has destroyed bacteria growing on a jellified medium.

plasmid
> A circular piece of DNA capable of self-replication within a cell independently of nuclear DNA. Frequently used as a vector (q.v.) in genetic engineering.

polymer
> A molecule made up of a number of smaller subunits.

polypeptide
> A stretch of amino acids constituting a protein or one chain (q.v.) of a multichain protein.

polyribosome

A collection of ribosomes (q.v.) attached to a messenger RNA molecule engaged in aiding the synthesis of proteins according to the coded instructions in the RNA.

primary transcript

That molecule of RNA first synthesized as a faithful copy of a whole gene when a gene is activated. Portions of the primary transcript are cut out before the messenger RNA moves to the cytoplasm.

probe

A stretch of DNA or RNA labelled with a radioactive isotope, capable of binding to, and thus 'finding' a stretch of DNA with a complementary sequence.

protein

Molecules composed of amino acids and which perform most of the cell's work. Includes enzymes, hormones, antibodies, carriers for other molecules, receptors and structural molecules.

protein kinase

An enzyme which catalyses the addition of a phosphate group to certain amino acids of proteins.

protein synthesis

The process by which the amino acids are joined together to form proteins. Almost synonymous with peptide synthesis, except that the latter usually refers to shorter stretches of amino acids.

restriction endonucleases

Enzymes which cut the DNA double helix only when a particular sequence of base pairs is present.

retrovirus

A virus which uses RNA as the genetic material but possesses the enzyme reverse transcriptase (q.v.) and which can thus cause a DNA copy of itself or some part of itself to be made inside the cell.

reverse transcriptase

An enzyme capable of using RNA as a template and creating a DNA copy of the relevant sequence.

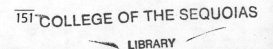

ribosomes

> Small, particulate entities within the cytoplasm which attach to messenger RNA and help to translate that message into a particular amino acid sequence. Essential for protein synthesis in the cell.

RNA

> Ribonucleic acid. A single-stranded molecule consisting of sugar, phosphate and a string of bases. Different sorts of RNA have different functions. Messenger RNA is the immediate template for protein synthesis.

sticky ends

> Short single-stranded sequences of DNA capable of binding to short, complementary stretches on other DNA molecules.

substrate

> The target for an enzyme's action.

Tay-Sachs disease

> An inherited disease, occurring predominantly in Ashkenazi Jews, due to a genetic defect in an enzyme, hexosaminidase A, which leads to abnormal accumulation of certain fats in nerve cells causing severe mental retardation and death.

thymine

> One of the small molecular building blocks called bases, which make up the coding units of DNA and RNA. Often abbreviated to T. In DNA, pairs with adenine (A).

tissue typing

> The process by which scientists determine the genes of a person which are important for organ transplantation.

transcription

> The process whereby the DNA double helix unwinds and an RNA copy of a gene is synthesized complementary to one of the strands.

transfection

> Insertion of DNA into a cell without a vector and integration of that DNA with the cell's own genes. Generally an inefficient process but occurs sufficiently frequently that, if transfected cells can be selectively grown, genetic engineering can be achieved.

transfer RNA

An abbreviation of amino acid transfer RNA. Each particular transfer RNA molecule can ferry a particular amino acid to the right spot on the ribosome, thus helping in protein synthesis.

translation

The process by which the coded message in messenger RNA is read, resulting in the formation of a corresponding protein.

transposons

Mobile stretches of DNA which can move around within the genome instead of (like most DNA) residing in one place in the one chromosome.

uracil

A base unique to RNA, informationally equivalent to cytosine in DNA. Abbreviated to U.

vaccine

A preparation used in the immunization of a person or animal, designed to protect the immunized individual from a particular virulent infection.

vacuole

A sack-like subcellular entity in a cell which looks relatively translucent in the electron microscope. Frequently involved in transporting food into the cell or some secreted product out of the cell.

vector

A tool of the genetic engineer used to transport recombinant DNA into a host cell and to permit its extensive replication there, independently of the replication of the cell's own DNA; a generic term covering phages, plasmids, cosmids and other types of mobile DNA.

virus

The smallest and simplest forms of life. Micro-organisms which are obligatory parasites, capable of multiplying only inside living cells.

Index

Words marked with an asterisk are included in the Glossary (pages 142 to 153).